SICKBED
TO SUMMITS

SICKBED TO SUMMITS

The Story of Triumph Over Adversity

SARA CROSLAND

ISBN: 979-8-6875-7300-9

Book design by Wordzworth
www.wordzworth.com

Published by Sara Crosland
www.saracrosland.com

"Sara has made an amazing recovery and has been a true inspiration to others since the surgery, in no small part because of her positive attitude and ability to keep going through adversity.

She has clearly demonstrated that whilst this type of surgery can be very challenging to recover from, with the right approach you can return to normal life.

Sara is an amazing role model to those having to go through similar treatment."

—PROFESSOR SIMON LLOYD
Consultant Neurotologist and Professor of Otolaryngology

After my diagnosis in January 2020, I joined BANA – The British Acoustic Neuroma Association. I came across Sara some months later, when she delivered an inspirational and thought-provoking presentation to the BANA annual conference.

Later, I was intrigued by the webinar Sara presented in her role of BANA ambassador. I knew this was a lady with a story to tell, one that was far from complete.

Sara has written a very personal account of her Acoustic Neuroma journey, quite literally taking the reader from sickbed to summits. Whilst this is the journey of a devastating, life changing diagnosis, it is also an account of how one individual rises to master physical and mental challenges.

This is an uncompromising account, sometimes sad, often funny, but always pragmatic. We see patient, wife, mum, photographer and adventurer as Sara shares the pain, and joy of life with an Acoustic Neuroma.

—HELEN BRIGGS

FOREWORD

Several years ago our path crossed with Sara's quite by chance. We got to know an optimistic educator, who had her mind set on pushing her limits, and as an athlete, she demonstrated just how dedicated she was to it.

As experts in pushing endurance limits, Sara came to us for advice and support in her efforts to do the same. Little did we know, that soon enough, she would be the one teaching us a lesson in determination.

In early 2018, Sara was diagnosed with an Acoustic Neuroma brain tumour. We remember the day she shared the news with us, and we were not overly surprised she took it as a challenge to overcome rather than the end of the world.

We are soldiers. Our true worth is measured only under extreme conditions, but Sara soon made us realize that the same goes for any man or woman and that the mindset of a warrior is not restricted to us military folk.

The pre-op Sara was a runner, a hiker, a violinist, and she had a keen eye for photography; all of this was in jeopardy, as she went under the knife. She bravely went through with it, knowing that her family and friends will have her back during recovery and a selection of US Navy men will push her to break her new set limits and pick her up when she's down.

Sure, there were low points. The loss of hearing in one ear, nausea, and the struggle to walk and keep her balance, all were expected of course but were hard to adjust to and deal with as they manifested.

We have seen our fair share of hurt brothers, and the common thing to them all was their eagerness to get back in the fight. That was exactly what we saw in post-op Sara, that internal fire to get back in the fight. She rode her bike and did yoga just weeks after surgery to teach her body balance again; she took long hikes, and conquered summits to let her body know that going back to what she was before the op was just the beginning.

For us here, it was no surprise that Sara rose to the challenge. It was impressive to watch, and an inspiration to us all, but we were most impressed by how she transformed her own experience to a newfound purpose, a calling to help and support others that went through or go through the same challenge, to share the healing magic of optimism and determination.

People often wonder why bad things happen to good people. After accompanying Sara through her ordeal we came to the conclusion, that in a twisted way, we are all lucky she went through this. We all received a role model to learn from and important lessons in optimism and mind over body.

E.N.B.
UNITED STATES NAVY

ACKNOWLEDGEMENTS

This book would not have been possible without the support of my friends and family.

First and foremost, I want to thank my husband and best friend, Neil. Thank you for supporting me and my dreams. You have been beside me through everything life has thrown at us and never flinched. You never tell me that I can't. You are my rock. My story is as much yours as it is mine, and I am thankful you have supported me in writing this story.

To my children, Olivia, Daniel and Alex. My love for you all brought me through some of the darkest times of my life. I hope this book lets you know just how much I love you, and how grateful I am that I am here to watch you continue to grow.

To my mum, thank you for supporting my family when I couldn't. Thank you for providing meals, keeping on top of the housework, and all the other things I couldn't do for myself.

To Hugo our dog, thank you for your unconditional love and affection, and keeping me company when I couldn't move off the sofa. You really are my shadow and have helped to fill the huge void that existed when Max left us.

I wish to express my utmost thanks to Mr Scott Rutherford, Prof. Simon Lloyd, Prof. Andrew King, Andrea Wadeson and Helen Entwistle and everyone else involved in my care at Salford Royal. Without a doubt, I wouldn't have been here to write this book if it weren't for your knowledge and expertise.

To Sahra, Wendy and Di, thank you so much for being there, for stepping up to the mark when others were nowhere to be seen. "True friends walk in when everyone else has walked out."

Thank you to Helen, Liam, Cerries, Chris, Emily, Sharon, Candy, Karen and Julie for your input and being the extra pairs of eyes I needed.

To Jude. Thank you so very much for giving me the push I needed and helping to make this happen. For the words of wisdom, the humour, and the feedback. This book would likely never have happened without your help! I will be forever grateful for your support in getting my words onto paper.

To my editor, Amanda Harman, thank you so much for your time and expertise, for your words of encouragement, and for looking after my work!

To the many friends I have made during the course of my journey from sickbed to summits, and those I have yet to meet, thank you for inspiring me. I dedicate this book to each and every individual fighting a battle of their own. The phrase, "I thought about quitting, but then remembered who was watching" rings very true. For you all, I promise to make each and every day count.

Finally, to my Navy friends… Well, what can I say? Thank you for being there during some of the darkest days of my life, for allowing me to vent (from a safe distance!) and helping to forge me into the fighter I needed to be to win this battle. The glimpse I have had into your world of special operations has made me the strong person I am today, able to push far beyond my limitations (self-imposed or otherwise), and breaking that glass ceiling society places on us. You have given me the confidence I need to get back out there and live life. I don't think you understand just how very thankful I am that you were around during this time. I am forever grateful that our paths crossed and I consider you all great mentors, leaders and most importantly, friends.

CHAPTER 1

Tuesday 20th February 2018 started off pretty much the same as any other day. I didn't feel great, but not feeling great was the new 'norm' for me: I hadn't felt great for a very long time. I was in the routine of pacing myself, so I could manage the constant levels of fatigue as best I could, and actually hide some of it from others. I'd been for an MRI (magnetic resonance image) scan on my brain that morning and had been a little concerned, because the nurse stopped the scan part way through in order to inject me with a contrast dye; I could see a cluster of people looking at the monitor, reflected in the mirror on the head coil I was wearing to help keep me still, but who knew if that was normal? I was suspicious.

I came home, sorted out the washing, and checked the kitchen cupboards, astounded as always at just how much food my very active teenagers got through – sometimes I thought we must have three extra people living in the house that I didn't know about. I made a mental note to pop into the supermarket later, and settled down to edit some photos I'd taken, as part of my new role as a portrait photographer. It was then I received a call from the hospital saying that they were sorry to have missed me, but the results from the MRI scan were in. Whilst I had an appointment arranged for the following week, the consultant apparently had a cancellation that afternoon. Could I pop back in to discuss them? I felt a little stab of irritation that I had to make the drive back there, as I was so tired, but I suppose these things happen. I confirmed that I would head straight back; at least I'd be able to do the food shopping on the way home.

I wasn't overly worried. I'd already had countless tests, all of which had revealed nothing untoward, other than a vitamin D deficiency, which is quite common given our lovely English weather and the general lack of sunshine. I was certain that this was another 'let's rule this out' exercise.

I drove myself to the hospital, eager to get the appointment over with, so I could get back to my photographs and carry on with my day. I met my specialist, who was exactly the same as he had been the week before; a larger-than-life character, bubbly and full of fun with a huge smile. I must have been a little tense, as I felt myself relax in the chair – surely this was a good sign, as he would be different if there was anything to worry about – there would be an atmosphere, or perhaps he'd be quite sombre, or there would be someone else in the room to deal with any upset.

"We found something this morning. We tried calling you back, but you'd already left the building." He beamed at me. "Do you want to see the image?"

Of course I wanted to see the image; it was the inside of my brain, and I'm a curious creature at the best of times – how many people get to see the inside of their brain? Plus, what had they found? He turned the portable screen towards me, so I could see the black-and-white image. It looked exactly the same as the ones I'd seen on the internet, except for one thing: a large white blob, situated to one side.

I was quite sure that wasn't supposed to be there. Instantly, I felt a flicker of fear.

"Well, what is it?" I asked, fighting down the growing sense of panic that was threatening to break forth at any second.

"We *think* it's a vestibular schwannoma." A what? That sounded like some exotic dish that you had with rice as a treat on a Saturday night. "We've already spoken to Walton Hospital, and an urgent referral has been made." Another smile. My brain made a couple of connections it didn't want to make. One, it was a brain tumour, and two, people died of brain tumours.

There is an expression, 'a gamut of emotions'. I can tell you that mine were gamutting all over the place. There were numbness, utter fear and anger all battling it out, with even a bit of relief that this was an actual thing, and as a thing, it had a name that I could identify with and deal with. Relief may appear to be a strange reaction, but there had been many months of feeling that there was something seriously wrong, but no firm answers. Although I didn't have a choice in the matter, my emotions eventually settled on anger.

"Well, what are you going to do about it? I still have things I need to do! I'm not ready to check out yet!"

"Oh, don't worry, it's treatable. Look, I'd like you to go back into the waiting room, and my colleague will come and speak to you in a few minutes." Another smile.

I was shocked beyond belief. Even if your brain flirts with the idea that it could be something as serious as this, you don't really believe it. You don't think that it could actually happen to you – this was a tragedy that happened to other people. People who were older. People who didn't take care of themselves. People who didn't have so much to live for. I gathered my belongings with shaking hands and made my way back to the waiting room, legs trembling with every step.

The room was small, hot, cramped and full of people. I sat in total silence, unable to control my shaking, and trying to focus on anything other than what was going on. I can still clearly recall the out-of-date popular magazines, the abandoned empty cups and the tea stains on the small coffee table. My husband, Neil, was on his way to meet me, but I needed some contact with him, there and then. I needed to tell him, as I couldn't cope with this on my own. With hands still trembling, I grabbed my phone and wrote, "There's something growing in my head that shouldn't be there." I couldn't bring myself to use the words brain tumour. Looking back, it was so selfish of me; I could and should have waited for him to arrive, but how on earth do you tell the one person you promised to spend the rest of your life with, the person you had so many plans with, the person that had sacrificed so much for both you and the family, that you have a brain tumour?

Of course, I did the one thing you're always told not to do, and I went straight to the internet. One of the first links to come up was a cancer charity website. Oh, wonderful! Not only a brain tumour, but now the word 'cancer' had joined in the party. I tried to concentrate on the 'treatable' bit, but it didn't help, as treatable is not the same as curable. I forced myself to click on the link.

A low-grade tumour, symptoms of vestibular schwannoma (sometimes referred to as acoustic neuroma) can be:

- Hearing loss that usually affects one ear

- Ringing and buzzing sounds in one or both ears (tinnitus)

- Difficulty working out where sounds are coming from

- Dizziness or vertigo

- Numbness of the face (this usually happens in advanced tumours)

Well, with the exception of the hearing loss, I could have written each and every one of the points made. In fact, to add an extra layer of excitement, I had one two more to add, including double vision on my left side. Acoustic neuromas are now thought to affect 1 in 50,000 people in the UK. To put that in perspective, there is a 0.002% chance of getting one, and yet here I was, one of the chosen ones. Why me? Why now?

I'd always been lucky. Exceptionally lucky. I was very happily married to my soul mate, who I'd met at quite a young age. I had three wonderful teenage children, who were approaching adulthood without too many bumps in the road. I had a strong family around me. I had a career in special needs education. I was a classical violinist. As any parent will tell you, years of juggling work, study and a young family are rewarding, but they're also extremely hard work. At 42, I'd reached the point in my life where the pressure was easing and there was a little more time just for Neil and me. I had taken the plunge and followed my dream of setting up a small portrait photography studio, which was building nicely and starting to flourish. I was embracing my love of the outdoors with running, hiking and my new-found hobby of climbing. I'd even grasped the opportunity to go paragliding in the Alps, and I'd loved every second. Suddenly, I realised that there were so many things that I still wanted to do, and I was making plans. Big plans. I was making things happen. I was excited, and looking forward to a future that appeared to be very bright indeed. It seemed so unfair that all of this was being snatched away. I looked at the people around me: they were old; they were sick and they were frightening. I didn't belong here – only I did, as I was sick too.

My present story had started many months before. Our beloved dog, Max, had reached the end of his journey and we'd made the hardest decision ever, but the best decision for him. The night before the vet's visit, dreading the loss of him, I laid on the floor and slept fitfully beside him, to prolong every minute that we had left together. A couple of days later, I began to experience pain in my joints, particularly my hips; I put it down to sleeping on the floor and life generally feeling a bit rubbish at that time. The pain didn't ease off, as I'd hoped, but radiated to my knees, my ankles, my feet, my elbows and my hands and fingers. It wasn't the sort of ache that you get with something like the flu; it was more severe and it wasn't getting any better.

I had also developed an unusual rash, which was painful rather than itchy. Over a few days, it seemed to fade away, then flare up again. I went to my GP, who sent me for the obligatory blood test. And another. And another. Eventually, the vitamin D deficiency showed up, which did match up with the aching joints and fatigue, and I thought we'd nailed it; boost my vitamin D levels and we'd be home and dry. Not so. My inflammatory markers were up, so with a diagnosis of polyarthralgia, the next step was extremely strong anti-inflammatory drugs to try to manage the symptoms at the very least. My body wasn't too happy with those, and protested with a persistent upset stomach. The pain was so severe, at one point I accidentally overdosed on red wine and ibuprofen, just to get some relief. Not to be recommended. I was constantly exhausted and nauseous, and I was tired of never feeling right. My social life had dwindled to practically nothing, as I tried to keep enough energy, just so I could make it into work, but even that had become a major struggle, resulting in me resigning from my role. Although people were lovely to my face, I could tell that they didn't understand and were getting fed up of what looked like a complete lack of effort on my part; if only they knew what it took to get up in the mornings.

Totally out of the blue, the pain began to recede. It didn't disappear, it just became more bearable, and I assumed that either the inflammation was settling down, or my pain threshold had increased. The exhaustion was still there though. At roughly the same time, I realised that my left cheek didn't feel right; not exactly numb, but there was a noticeable and strange sensation. I also developed a touch of double vision and tinnitus, but as a classical musician, who had played with orchestras, tinnitus can be part of the territory. I went back to the GP, with a 'sorry, it's me again' attitude, and wondering if I was going to end up with my own chair in the waiting room, and a small but tasteful brass plaque to commemorate the occasion of the most appointments ever. My GP immediately told me that she was concerned about the neurological symptoms. The previous year, I had suffered a tick bite, which can lead to Lyme disease, and this along with MS (multiple sclerosis) was now on the radar. Whilst I sat there, she spoke to a neurologist and I was admitted to hospital on the same day for tests, including an MRI scan and a lumbar puncture. Things had turned serious very quickly indeed. I'm not sure why, but the MRI scan and the lumbar puncture didn't actually take place at that time, but an absolute barrage of other tests did. The MRI was scheduled for the following week, which is why I now found myself sitting in that waiting room.

It probably wasn't very long, but it felt like forever before I was called back into the office to see another consultant. I'd never met him before, but he looked very serious, slightly disorganised and almost flustered, which was obviously not his natural state. You and me both, buddy. With hindsight, I think this was probably a rarity for him and one of the very, very few occasions where he was dealing with such a diagnosis; or maybe he'd been warned that I was seriously unhappy with the situation, and possibly quite scary. He may have needed a hard hat and armoured vest at that point. The portable computer screen had gone, and he began to explain the next steps. At that point, Neil was shown in, and I nearly lost it completely. He was visibly shaken and upset, and just for a second, I saw my own fears and panic reflected in his eyes before he shut it down and replaced it with neutrality. A new and very powerful emotion entered the ring: guilt. Oh, how could I put my loved ones through this? There was nothing I could say or do to make it any better or take away the fear that was swamping both of us.

The consultant decided that a matter-of-fact approach was the best way forward, and he began to explain the MRI results to Neil, who remained silent and motionless. He explained that an urgent referral had been made to the local neurological centre, and I should soon hear from them. He then asked how I'd got to the hospital, which I thought was an odd change of subject, but I told him that I'd driven in my car. He asked us to wait, while he contacted the DVLA to see if I was still allowed to drive. Allowed to drive? What? Oh no, they couldn't take my licence off me. Not here. Not now. I'd walked in here less than an hour ago, with a relatively normal life, and now it was being dismantled before my eyes. No car meant severely restricted independence. How would I run the children about to their jobs, friends and clubs? How would I get to my studio to earn my living? How would I do the shopping? How would I get to appointments? How would I meet friends for coffee? All of these are totally trivial in the grand scheme of things, but at that moment in time, they were everything. My thoughts whirled around uncontrollably, as Neil and I stood in a busy corridor, in our own bubble of weirdness. Another little thought crept forward – if I didn't make it through this, and there was no guarantee I would, I wouldn't need a car anyway.

"You're ok to continue driving," confirmed the consultant when he returned. "You're free to go home," he added, "but if you experience any worsening of symptoms, or a sudden headache, you must come straight back to the emergency department". There was something about his tone that underlined the seriousness of his words. Was this thing unstable then? Could I collapse in a heap at any moment? Common sense told me that it was unlikely, as they'd allowed me to drive, but once the thought was there, it was there.

Neil's warm hand slid over my cold one, and gently squeezed it. That squeeze and the expression in his eyes told me that he would be there, no matter what, as he always had been. I'd been fighting back the tears every step of the way, but now I could feel them welling up again with such force, there was no ignoring them.

"I'll drive and we'll sort out getting your car later," Neil mumbled. He led me through the hospital corridors, still holding my hand, as though I were a child. I was happy to let him, as I don't think I could have found my way out alone. I felt fragile and broken. Everything was a blur. Once I was in the car, the crying started in earnest; Niagara Falls had nothing on me that day.

"What am I going to say to my mum? And what about the children?" I cried. Daniel had his exams that summer. Alex had just started Year 10 and was working towards his GCSEs. How could they achieve their best under these horrific circumstances? I knew I couldn't tell them. My mind raced as I started to think of ways that perhaps I could have the treatment, whatever that might be, on the quiet. Scheduling hospital appointments for school hours. Having treatments when there were fewer people around, so no one could let the secret out. Finding excuses to cover up the side effects. I was strong. Surely I could disguise anything?

It was impossible, and I knew it, but I also knew that I needed to try anything and everything to protect as many people as possible. I wasn't prepared for the feelings of extreme embarrassment, or the shame of the upset that I was about to unleash upon everyone. It felt as though I had committed some egregious crime – I alone was to shoulder the blame, it was all my fault; I was responsible for this mess and there was nothing I could do about it. How could I let this happen? As we sat at the traffic lights, I watched people walking by, talking, laughing and enjoying themselves, and I found it difficult to understand how their world continued to turn, whilst mine and everything I knew crumbled around me. It was a low point, for sure.

Once we got home, I went back to the computer and to the photographs I was editing. I wanted to immerse myself in work, to forget the horror of what was going on, but all I could do was stare blankly at the screen. No matter how hard I tried, I just couldn't do it. Nothing made sense anymore, and as the frustration grew, so did the tears. What did I say about Niagara Falls? Neil had decided that our parents needed to know, and he had gone to tell them face to face. I didn't agree, but I didn't have strength to argue – deep down, I knew he was right and I would just have to dig deep and find a way of dealing with the guilt and shame of causing so much upset. It wasn't long until he was back, with everyone in tow, which was unexpected and unwanted.

Suddenly, well-meaning experts remarking, "They'll be able to sort it out," and "Everything will be ok," surrounded me. If anyone had said, "These things happen for a reason," I may well have throttled them with my bare hands. I found myself nodding in agreement, even though the tears were just seconds away, and I really wanted to scream with frustration. I know their words came from the heart and they were only trying to take my pain away, in the same way that I would have done anything not to cause it. Nobody knew if they could sort it out, and even if they could, what treatment was it going to be and how was I going to be at the end of it? The terror of the enormity of the situation was growing with every passing moment. I know it's an awful thing to say, but I was relieved when they left and I could drop the pretence. I needed time. Time to think. Time to plan. Time to find me again, even though I had no idea who this new me would be. One thing that I did absolutely insist on was that no one told our children exactly what was happening. They knew I hadn't been well and they were far from stupid, so we decided to downplay things and tell them that I had a problem with a nerve in my head, which may need an operation at some stage to correct it. We then did a 'business as usual' approach, with such good acting skills – if there are any Oscars going spare, I have a well-polished shelf that they'd look particularly good on.

Looking back, it was part coping-mechanism and part denial. Oh, and something else had arrived, opened a packet of biscuits and made itself at home: Doubt. Now, I'd met Doubt previously, as everyone has, but he'd never stuck round for long. Generally, I'm a very determined and positive person; I view obstacles as challenges to be overcome, rather than permanent barriers.

Doubt was different this time, though, and I knew he was going to be difficult to shift; there was quite a confident air to him, and he'd even brought his slippers.

The following weeks were very strange indeed. On the surface, life continued as normal and yet this huge unknown thing that we couldn't really talk about was hanging over us. I would wake in the middle of the night, consumed by fear and panic. Sometimes I would wake in the morning, and for a few seconds everything would feel ok, until the realisation swept over me with a force that took my breath away. Every single day, apart from Sundays, I waited for the news of the urgent hospital referral; every letter, every phone call, every text…and yet there was nothing. Our lives were on hold. Doubt made his presence known on a regular basis. Neil was feeling particularly frustrated with the situation and had taken to researching every bit of information that he could, with a 'knowledge is power' approach – I understood: doing something useful was his coping mechanism.

He found a specialist that really caught his attention, a neurosurgeon based at Salford Royal in Manchester, which is relatively close to where we live. He was mentioned so often I began to think that he was part of the household. We were lucky enough to secure an urgent appointment with said Mr Scott Rutherford.

As we sat in the waiting area outside his office, *Back to Black* by Amy Winehouse played quietly on the radio. I sang along silently to myself, but its minor key and lyrics did little to lift my mood – there's a lot of 'goodbyes' and 'died' in that song, I'll have you know. Once again, it felt as though time had stopped, until we were called in. And that was when I felt that my luck might have improved, slightly. You know when you just take to someone on sight, and you like them and trust them instantly? That was the case with Mr Rutherford. Our local hospital had promised to send the MRI scan results across, but they didn't arrive in time for our appointment. As we had no images, Mr Rutherford asked me to explain what I had been shown, and I talked about the large white blob, as best I could. I think he was a little dubious when I said about the size of it, but nevertheless, he went on to break down the myths about vestibular schwannomas. Oh, the relief to listen to that calm, reassuring voice of reason, laying the facts out, one by one, and displaying obvious expertise.

He began to explain the treatment options: if it wasn't causing any symptoms, and was a small, slow-growing variety or stable, then the preferred option was watch and wait. Surprisingly, that didn't actually appeal to me. I felt as though I had an intruder in my head, and I just wanted it gone, never to think of it, or to worry about it again.

If the tumour were found to be growing more rapidly, then the next option would be radiation treatment. This treatment goes under various names that sound as though they could be hard rock bands: stereotactic radiosurgery, cyber and gamma knife, to name a few. They all work on the principle of a single high dose of radiation. It can take months to discover if this method has been successful, with the tumour often swelling and causing a worsening of symptoms before it stops growing, begins to shrink, or dies off. Funnily enough, this option didn't sound too appealing either.

The final possibility is based on the size of the tumour. Once it has reached a certain size, the only option is surgery. This would be using a translabyrinthine (rock band) approach, removing part of the skull behind the ear, accessing the tumour, debulking it, and then picking it away from the surrounding cranial nerves. Another attractive approach – not.

Vestibular schwannomas grow on the eighth cranial nerve, the vestibulocochlear (hearing and balance) nerve. Unfortunately, this means that they are in very close proximity to the facial and trigeminal nerves, which can be damaged during surgery. Calmly, Mr Rutherford explained the likelihood of the various side effects of surgery, none of which I wanted to hear: hearing loss, loss of balance, facial paralysis, difficulty swallowing, tinnitus, double vision, headaches, fatigue… the words rolled on – how's that for a veritable picnic of terrifying possibilities? "But," he added, "let's wait until I've seen your images, and then we'll have a better idea of what is going on. These tumours are slow growing, so we do have time on our side and don't have to rush any decisions in terms of treatment". The thing was, I did want to rush. I wanted this 'thing' out of my head and I wanted it out as soon as possible. I wanted my life back, or as much of it as I could possibly get back, as enough had been stolen from me as it was. I think Mr Rutherford was slightly taken aback by my attitude; he must have been used to people who were desperate to avoid surgery and yet here I was, almost pushing for it. I'm not saying that I was desperate, but if he'd have offered to operate there and then on his desk, with just a whiff of anaesthetic and a rusty pen knife, it wouldn't have been an outright no from me…

Finally, he carried out a few tests on my balance: I stood there, doing my best to follow various instructions. Some I could do and some I had difficulty with. He also examined my eyes and told me that I was suffering from nystagmus, an involuntary eye movement, and that could explain some of the vertigo-like symptoms I'd been experiencing. He also said that he would call me, as soon as he'd had sight of my MRI scans. I left the appointment feeling surprisingly calm and satisfied that although I'd heard a lot of things that weren't particularly thrilling we'd made progress.

True to his word, Mr Rutherford saw the scans and called me the following day. Neil and I sat upstairs, with the phone on loudspeaker. He confirmed that it did indeed look like a vestibular schwannoma, and that it was 3.5 cm in diameter, which was considered to be at the larger end of the scale. He told me that having had sight of the MRI scan, it was apparent that we had an added complication in that the tumour was cystic, which meant that whilst usually slow growing, cystic tumours can behave unpredictably, with the cysts often growing faster than the tumour itself, taking up valuable room in a confined space.

The MRI had also shown that my brainstem, which would normally look quite symmetrical on the images, was now becoming compressed. Whilst he had originally said that we had time on our side, he now felt that it would need to be treated sooner, rather than later, and that meant surgery. As I had been expecting the call, I'd prepared a list of questions, which was now held in a trembling, clammy hand. My first and most important question was that if I were to have surgery sooner, would my hearing on that side be salvaged? My little spurt of hope was dashed, as the answer was a definite no. My hearing and balance nerve would be severed to access the tumour, and there would be no hope of saving any hearing on that side. In its simplest terms, if I wanted to increase the chances of saving my face, I had no choice but to sacrifice my hearing. For a violinist, that news was utterly devastating. When I heard those words, and knew that surgery was my only option, I couldn't deal with it at that moment, and I left the room, leaving Neil to handle the rest of the call.

In the weeks that followed, I desperately tried to keep doing 'business as usual'. Life became a juggling act of running the home, working in the studio as best I could and putting on a cheerful front, telling everyone that I was OK. Oh, and the hospital appointments; I was either waiting for an appointment, attending an appointment or waiting for results from an appointment, together with all of the associated stress. There were so many appointments. In some respects, it was good to be busy. It was essential to keep everything as normal as possible for the children, so I couldn't dwell or openly worry, although Doubt was waving at me on a regular basis, just to let me know that he was still there. Photography was an excellent distraction that gave me something to enjoy and get lost in. The hospital appointments gave me the sense that the intruder was being dealt with and its days were numbered. Was I coping? I'm really not sure; if there's something beyond fingertips, that's what I was hanging on by.

A few weeks later, it was my birthday, and Doubt brought me a present that I really didn't want, a host of dark thoughts. I didn't feel that I had anything to celebrate. This could potentially be my last birthday with full facial movement. It would definitely be my last birthday with full hearing. It could even be my last birthday full stop. My future was far from certain. I was terrified. I just wanted to close my eyes and wake up in the best possible shape, when everything was over.

In an effort to cheer myself up. I treated myself to a trip to the hair salon, which wasn't really the treat I was hoping for. With the threat of potential facial paralysis looming, I ended up discussing styles that would cover the damaged areas of my face with Nicky, my stylist. She was wonderful and suggested a graduated bob, parted in such a way that the hair would fall across the bad side, and possibly a vivid colour to draw the eye away from my face; I was toying with the idea of bright purple. Surely that would be attention-grabbing enough? I sat there, looking at my reflection, whilst Nicky held my hair in a simulated bob so I could see what it looked like, and she told me that it would be so easy to handle, it would dry quickly and it would be cooler in hot weather; I didn't want to know. I don't think anyone appreciates just how much your face and hair can form part of your identity, until you are at risk of losing them. I have had long hair for as long as I can remember, because I love my long hair. Neil fell in love with me with long hair and yet here I was, with half my face covered, as though I was peering from behind a curtain. Don't get me wrong, the style was lovely, and there are many people who have to lose all of their hair for so many reasons, who would kill to have the choice of a bob, but the thought of having to make yet another forced and unwanted decision was devastating to me. I'm not ashamed to admit that I cried.

Later that day, I received a message from some good friends serving in the US Navy, who at that time were based somewhere out in the Middle East. They messaged to wish me a happy birthday and asked about my birthday plans. I don't know if it was the timing, if it was just because it was the written word, or if it was because of who it was, but the front I had so carefully maintained for weeks, crumbled. I told them that I wasn't doing anything. I told them that I felt utterly rubbish and didn't want to do anything. I told them that I just didn't want to acknowledge the fact that it could be my last birthday. If I was expecting sympathy, I was going to be disappointed. I was told in no uncertain terms that I needed to stop myself from having such morbid thoughts. Easy for them to say! They then went on to tell me a story that their chief would tell them, whenever they had morbid thoughts. I had the impression that given their situation, morbid thoughts were a genuine thing. The story they told went something like this:

There was a rich merchant somewhere in Baghdad who had a few stands in the local market. One day, one of his employees saw a suspicious figure walking around the market with a black hood, skeletal face with glowing red eyes, holding a scythe and asking questions. When the scary dude reached the terrified employee he asked, "Are you Abdullah Ibrahim Mansur?" The employee waved his hand (even though he was Abdullah Ibrahim Mansur), dropped everything and ran to his merchant boss. When he got to his boss, he told him everything that had happened and asked for the fastest horse the merchant had, so he could flee as far as he could from the Grim Reaper. The merchant gave the poor guy a horse and went to replace him at the market stand. As soon as he arrived at the market, he immediately saw the Grim Reaper wandering around, so he grabbed him by the collar and asked, "What do you want with Abdullah? Don't you have anything better to do than scare my employees?" Grim Reaper replied, "I wasn't trying to scare him. I was just very surprised to see him here. It's not his time... I have a meeting with him 3,000 miles from here in Samarra tomorrow."

The point of this story is that we will die when we die. Thinking about it won't change anything. We can't do anything about it. So, with that in mind, we should live well whilst we're alive, and not live our lives in fear of death, because that does nothing but screw up living. Their words hit home. I owe these guys so much. Despite the fact it was the last thing I felt like doing, I dressed up, put a smile on my face, and I went out to celebrate my birthday. OK, it wasn't the best evening of my life, but I did enjoy it more than I would have thought possible.

My thoughts kept returning to the Samarra tale. My Navy friends have a knack of giving me a psychological shove in the right direction when I need it, and I really needed it. I have always been a huge fan of to-do lists and goals, but maybe I needed to extend that and set myself some firm targets. Actually, some really tough firm targets, to make it worthwhile. I looked around for anything suitable and found the details of the Race for Life, but it was only 4 months later, on 8th July. I had no idea what state I would be in at that point. Would I have even had my surgery? Unknown. The uncertainties of the next few months were adding to the anger and frustration. I needed things to focus on, so I could feel as though I had some control over my life. To hell with it… I'd crawl, if I had to! Entered.

I moved on. What had I always wanted to do, but not achieved as yet? The Three Peaks Challenge for one, and climbing Jebel Toubkal, the highest peak in the Atlas Mountains, for another. At this point, I had a bit of a wobble and Doubt took full advantage. Why had these stayed only as a dream? Why hadn't I just done them when I had the chance? There were a few answers to that, but the main one was that I thought I had time, plenty of time. Now I didn't know what state I was going to be in after the surgery, or if it would be possible. Anger surfaced once again; I really was turning into Little Miss Furious these days and the temptation to stamp my foot was getting ever stronger. I gave Doubt a shove out of the way. To hell with it; they both went on the list, although I did acknowledge to myself that these were targets for some time in the future…well, at least more than four months away, anyway.

The next stage involved further discussions with Mr Rutherford about the preparation for surgery. He had a suggestion that made my toes curl, and not in a good way. He suggested a series of intratympanic gentamicin injections, a relatively new treatment for balance problems. These little darlings are a course of injections, directly into the inner ear, and no, you're not unconscious for it. The theory is that gentamicin is an antibiotic, but in high doses it can be ototoxic, which means toxic to the ear. It can cause damage to the mechanisms of hearing and balance within the ear. Usually, that's not a desirable outcome, but in my case, the plan was to slowly take away the balance function, on the basis that my brain would learn to compensate prior to surgery, and this would shorten my recovery time; I wouldn't be healing from major brain surgery and dealing with huge balance issues at the same time. Oh, wasn't I the lucky one? Right, for anyone who has the option to have these injections, I can't lie – they weren't particularly pleasant, but I personally believe they're worth every second of it, even if you just get a little post-op help from them. Anything that helps on that side of things is worth it.

Once the treatment started, my symptoms worsened considerably, in part due to the effects of the gentamicin but also, I suspect, because of the growing tumour or cysts pressing on my brainstem. To begin with, there were some small changes. My hearing, which had been absolutely fine, would intermittently worsen. I was in the car when I first noticed it, as I had to turn up the volume on the passenger side speakers, so that the sound was balanced for me. Some sounds were slightly distorted, sounding like an irritating, tinny speaker, and I was struggling to hear the high frequencies that I'd never had difficulty with previously. Just for an extra delight, the effects of my tinnitus really ramped up, reminding me of Prosecco fizzing in a glass; cruel, in more ways than one.

There were bigger and more worrying changes too. I rapidly lost a significant amount of balance, which caused me some crashing lows and Doubt to do a dance of delight. On one occasion, I just needed a break from everything and I'd arranged to meet a friend for coffee at a local garden centre. I'd driven there and was quite excited to have a long overdue catch-up; to relax and just have a laugh with a good friend. As I got out of my car, the lack of balance hit and I staggered across the car park, almost bumping into another customer. As I went to apologise, he snarled, "Put more water in it". It was the first time I'd personally experienced some of the ignorance that surrounds a hidden disability. I was mortified. I tried to laugh it off, but inside I was torn between wanting to cry and wanting to punch him, hard, if I could have kept my balance long enough to make it count. This incident really upset me and triggered the very real fear that someone could report me for drink driving; the thought of being stopped and breathalysed on the side of the road, in front of everyone, and no one listening to the fact I had a brain tumour, was too much to bear. Much to Doubt's delight, I made the decision to stop driving. I had no idea how emotionally vulnerable I was at that stage.

Before I go into the nitty-gritty of what happened next, I want you to know that I thought long and hard about whether to write this at all. If someone is newly diagnosed with a vestibular schwannoma and is looking to this as a source of comfort, it's not going to happen in this chapter. The thing to remember is that the vast majority of people who are diagnosed will not have a journey like mine. A number of factors worked against me: I had the late onset of symptoms and no hearing loss, which led to a late diagnosis. My tumour was already at 3.5 cm before it made itself known, which meant that the majority of options had already been stripped away from me. My tumour was cystic,

19

which made it unstable, and it was that instability that caused additional issues. My problem is that if you don't understand the lows, you can't appreciate the highs – what exactly is possible with the right mindset (as well as a great medical team and terrific support from family and friends). The consensus of opinion is that you need all of the detail, so here it is.

As if I wasn't going through enough, the nausea I'd been feeling for some weeks turned into actual vomiting; I really wasn't a fan of that. On the basis that it was potentially caused by vertigo, I was prescribed Prochlorperazine to help with the dizziness and Ondansertron and Hyoscine patches to help with the sickness. I wasn't quite rattling, but not far off. Although this is successful for many people, none of it seemed to help me. I also began to suffer with bouts of hiccups. Nothing would stop them, and they certainly didn't help the feelings of nausea. With every day that went by, I honestly felt as though the tumour was stripping layers of me away – more layers than I could have imagined. What would happen when there was nothing left?

Despite my best efforts, I became very weak, very quickly. The 'business as usual' approach was impossible to keep up, as I could barely move without being sick, and that's kind of difficult to disguise. With breaking hearts, we made the decision to tell the children exactly what was going on; a conversation that no parent should need to have. As Doubt kindly pointed out, they needed time to prepare, just in case I croaked. They were all amazing and incredibly resilient, each doing their best to help, in their own way. Before leaving for school each day, my youngest would hear me throwing up, as I lay in bed unable to make it to the bathroom, or even move. He would quietly come into the room, remove the sick bags, and return with a cup of tea and a piece of toast, telling me I'd feel so much better if I ate something, in exactly the same way as I'd said it to him as a small child. My children were 19, 16 and 14. They should never have had to see me in such a state. We are immensely proud of them.

My life had changed beyond recognition. I wasn't living anymore; I was merely existing. My mum had been an absolute godsend and I will never be able to thank her enough. Every single day, she turned up, did the housework, sorted the laundry and then cooked wonderful meals for all of us. She was warm, reassuring and provided as much support as she possibly could, particularly for the children. All I could do was lie on the sofa with our other dog Hugo, who wouldn't leave my side, with a sick bag in my hand, feeling utterly wretched and a failure. Doubt was almost purring with satisfaction.

The tumour was now affecting my taste buds, removing my ability to taste just about anything. I existed on water and mints, which was all I could tolerate for most of the time. My sense of smell was also affected. I kept thinking that something was burning, to the point where I was wondering if I'd had some form of supernatural experience; my grandmother, who I had been very close to before she died, had been a smoker and perhaps the smell was a sign that she had visited me; although I no longer believed in such things, it brought me some comfort. One of the most distressing things was the fact that I thought I smelled awful, and despite Neil's constant reassurances that I didn't, I always felt as though I needed to shower; not ideal when you can barely walk, never mind stand. As soon as Neil came home from work, he would help me into the shower and I would sit on the floor, feeling utterly sick and crying the whole time. If you want to know what broken looks like, that was it.

The simplest of daily tasks that everyone takes for granted became impossible. I found myself reaching for the same clothes day in, day out, as I couldn't work out what matched and what didn't. I couldn't think logically: my thought processes were tangled and it was exhausting to try and straighten them out. Even my handwriting was affected; no matter how hard I concentrated or how much effort I put into it, it came out resembling a toddler's scrawl and was usually illegible.

There were worrying physical symptoms too. My resting heart rate was usually around a respectable rate of 50–60 beats per minute, as my cardiovascular fitness was quite good from running and hiking; it was now almost double that, at 110. I was so angry that all this was happening to me, and I had absolutely no control over any of it. It was all so unfair.

Just when I didn't think I could cope with another single thing, Doubt really upped his game and went for the jugular. I began to wonder if I could hang on to life long enough to actually have the surgery – would I be physically strong enough to take it? It was bizarre that it was impossible to think logically about day-to-day things, but anything to do with death was crystal clear.

I received so many well-meaning, positive messages such as "Keep fighting," and "You've got this," which are obviously the natural things to say to someone in my position. I would have no doubt used them myself to someone else in the same position, but those words began to grate on me; they became a source of major irritation. People just don't realise what it's like to have been strong, fit and healthy, and to have that squeezed out of you, with each passing day. It's no exaggeration to say there were days where I wanted to go to sleep and never wake up. Sometimes, I would close my eyes, and a dream would appear of being out in the mountains somewhere, breathing in the crisp, clean air and enjoying the spectacular views, but the world I was now in couldn't have been further away. Physically and psychologically, I didn't know how much more I could take.

CHAPTER 2

Just over three weeks before my surgery, I had a rare good day, although by good day, I mean one that wasn't quite as bad as the others. Although I still felt nauseous, I'd stopped throwing up so much, and that made a world of difference to me. I'm sure you all must have had a sickness bug or eaten something that didn't agree with you, and experienced how much it knocks you about, even after a few days; well that was my permanent state. It was such a glorious Friday and I just wanted to feel the warmth of the sunshine on my skin. I made it outside, into a chair in the garden, sunglasses firmly in place, and felt myself begin to relax in what felt like the first time in forever. I'm not sure if I dozed off, but the ringing of my phone startled me; very few people contacted me for nice things these days. It was Di, a former colleague and a very good friend indeed. "What are you up to?" she asked. I explained that it was a better day, and although I still felt very nauseous and exhausted, I had made it out into the garden.

"Great!" she said "I'll come and get you at lunch time. You can pop into school and see everyone." I protested that I was too poorly to do it, but Di was having none of it. In the nicest possible way, she has the knack of making sure that you can't say no and an attitude of "What's a bit of sick between friends?" My brain said, "No way, we're not well enough and we can't be bothered." Doubt rolled around the floor pointing and laughing. My mouth said, "Yes".

In all honesty, I was glad of the distraction. It would be so lovely to see everyone again, as there hadn't been the chance to say a proper goodbye; plus I missed everyone. The thought of familiar people and surroundings, the warmth I associated with the place and some normal conversation about things other than my health, lifted my spirits in a way I thought was no longer possible. True to her word, Di arrived to collect me and we made what felt like a marathon journey to the car. When we got to the school, Di instinctively knew what to do, tucking her arm through mine in a friendly fashion, rather than thinking, "If I don't do this, she'll probably face plant and be a nuisance". We made our way through to the quad, where on fine days we usually sat for lunch. There were a couple of people who I really liked there, tucking into their food, and I sat down with them, while Di went to the staffroom to collect her lunch.

One of them, Carol, made me very welcome. She said how lovely it was to see me, and asked how I was doing, with genuine interest and concern. The other didn't even look up from her phone. She never said a word, completely ignoring my attempts to start a conversation. Di returned, having witnessed this from the staffroom, and picking up on my uncertainty and discomfort, suggested we sat elsewhere; to my extreme embarrassment, she had to help me to my feet and support me as we moved. This was the first time I'd experienced a total change of attitude in someone I liked and cared for; actually, someone I really admired and respected. Sadly, it wasn't the last, and Doubt had a field day with that. At the time, the rejection hurt like hell and I had little to no coping mechanism to deal with it. Now, I don't know; maybe people thought a brain tumour was contagious, or maybe I wasn't useful anymore, or maybe they weren't the people I thought they were in the first place. Perhaps they just didn't know how to respond. What were they expecting to see? A lump on my head? Serious illness is a great leveller. It's quite strange how people react to you; some of the people I thought would be there for me 100%, as I would have been for them, just disappeared. On the other hand, some of the most terrific support came from people I hardly knew. There's a saying that true friends walk in, when everyone else has walked out; I feel there's a lot of truth in that.

Another thing that was thrust into the fore was our financial situation, as our income had unexpectedly dropped and thrown a curve ball into our plans; I was watching my savings dwindle at an alarming rate, as I still had all of my studio outgoings, even though I wasn't making a penny. I had also been told that I shouldn't work for 12–16 weeks after surgery, due to the risks involved. Neil had told me not to worry and he was willing to step into the breach, but I still had the last tattered remnants of my pride; I'd signed the paperwork, it was my responsibility. In addition, Doubt had pointed out that if I were to die, Neil would be needing every penny he could get. My friend, Sahra had tentatively suggested that I apply for the financial assistance that she was convinced I was entitled to. Although I didn't want to go down this route for support, it was the most sensible solution. Sahra offered to help me with the paperwork on the Saturday, a gesture I was so grateful for, as I knew my poor befuddled brain and dodgy eyesight would not have been able to cope with it, and I really didn't want to have to ask Neil to deal with this on top of everything else.

In the early hours of Saturday morning, a raging headache woke me up. Determined not to wake Neil, who was probably as exhausted as I was, I took some of my ever-present painkillers and waited for them to take the edge off it. The headache was so severe it was causing a different type of nausea to the norm; who knew you could get different types of nausea? My head felt different; it felt as though half of my skull was filled with a really unpleasant, whooshing sensation. I closed my eyes, not wanting to stare into the blackness. Doubt appeared with a "Do you think…?" but I swatted him away; I really wasn't in the mood to deal with him at that moment. It took a long time to drift off into a disturbed sleep.

When I woke again, later that morning, I felt even worse. The sun was shining outside, but I couldn't bear it. I pulled the sheet over my head, not wanting to move, as the nausea was so severe. The exhaustion was excelling itself too, but I put that down to a busier-than-usual few days; I'd been to Manchester for my final gentamicin injection, taken part in a research project that was examining the way in which acoustic neuromas grow, and I'd also had that afternoon at school. All that, together with the upset it had caused me doesn't sound much, but given the state I was in, it took all the energy I had. Time felt as though it had slowed right down and I felt incredibly sluggish and disorientated. Little did I know what was really going on. Mum called in that morning, popped her head around the bedroom door to see how I was, and tried to cajole me into getting up and dressed.

"I'll get up soon," I mumbled, trying to appease her.

Eventually, I dragged myself out of bed. By now it was lunchtime, and as I couldn't stand the thought or smell of food, I took myself off to sit under the parasol outside. Even with my sunglasses on, it was still too bright. I closed my eyes and fell asleep once more. I woke shortly before Sahra arrived and we made a start on the long-winded and complicated application form for personal independence payments. The near constant headache that I'd had for weeks was becoming unbearable again; I thought it was due to the bright sunshine, and the effort of struggling to think clearly on the most basic details of my life to complete the form. As I was struggling with the brightness, we moved inside.

I remember Sahra talking me through each section of the form, correcting my usually perfect spelling, whilst I tried to make notes in my childish scrawl for what needed to be completed. I was finding it impossible to concentrate. The pain in my head was all-consuming. I finally reached the point where I couldn't take any more. I remember saying, "I'm sorry, can we do this another day? I'm really not feeling too good.". Sahra was amazing, as always, completely understood and left immediately. Almost as soon as Neil closed the door behind her, I had the most excruciating pain in my head and neck, far worse than I had previously experienced. The only way to describe it is how I would imagine it must feel to be clobbered around the back of the head, with a sizeable plank of wood, and with considerable force. Without warning, I was violently sick.

"This isn't right," I sobbed to Neil. He wanted to take me to hospital straight away, but it was a Saturday evening and I was terrified of waiting in a busy emergency department, clogged up with people who'd been drinking all day in the sunshine, and who were now suffering as a result of it.

"I don't want to go," I told him. I knew I wasn't being at all rational, but I couldn't help it. There was a full-on war going on in my head. I wanted to curl up in a ball on the sofa and ignore everything, but I just knew something was very seriously wrong. I'd been trained in emergency first aid and knew that if this had happened to someone else in my presence, by now they'd either be halfway to hospital in my car, or we'd be waiting for an ambulance, and I wouldn't have taken no for an answer; when it's you though, it's different.

Neil was torn. He knew I desperately needed to go to hospital, but he was worried about upsetting me any further and making things worse. It was a delicate balancing act.

"Look…" he said. "We'll just go along to the hospital and see what they say…" The pain kicked up another notch, and I don't think I even replied. We grabbed my hospital paperwork and my emergency kit of multiple sick bags and kitchen roll, and drove the 6 miles to hospital, very quickly indeed. Once there, I was barely able to stand unaided, so I sat down whilst Neil registered my details at the reception desk, telling them that I had a brain tumour.

"Take a number and wait to be seen by triage," came the somewhat unconcerned reply.

By this point, I could barely speak because of the pain; it was a relentless pounding, deep inside my skull and there was no escape from it. I felt so sick, but thankfully I'd not eaten that day so I just sat there, retching every few minutes. People looked over, as mindless Saturday night TV shows, full of canned laughter, blared from the screen above my head. I must have looked ridiculous, sitting there with my head in my hands, wearing sunglasses as I still couldn't stand the bright lights. If someone had given me the option to die quietly there and then, I might have been tempted.

It was some 40 minutes before we were called through to triage. As Neil tried to explain my condition, the nurse took my pulse and blood pressure. Both were high, as I expected. Then she looked at my pupils.

"Is your left pupil normally dilated?" she asked, showing a mild curiosity. No, of course it bloody wasn't. I felt angry and irritable. I was asked to take a seat back in the waiting room, whilst they tried to find me a side room with dimmable lights. It was about another 15 minutes before we were taken through. Neil was shocked. He had only wanted us to be given advice, and really wasn't expecting this. We were both completely out of our depth. I lay down on the patient trolley, and the lights were dimmed to a point that was just about bearable. The nurses had realised the severity of what was going on and tried to manage my pain, with intravenous paracetamol and morphine, along with anti-sickness medication. Nothing worked. The pain was excruciating. Even Doubt looked a bit worried.

Sometime later, I was taken to have a CT (computerised tomography) scan. The porter who wheeled me there was lovely, and so kind; I must have appeared plain rude, as I just couldn't speak because of the pain. The back of my head felt like it was clamped in an ever-tightening vice, and I really didn't want to lie in the scanner. It must only have taken minutes, and before I knew it, I was back in the side room with Neil. People quietly came and went, checking my vital signs, looking at the drips, and asking how my pain levels were. I told Neil to go home as he was completely exhausted, but he refused point blank to leave me. Eventually, he fell asleep resting on me, and I listened to his breathing, glad that he had at least a few minutes of respite from the nightmare we were in; it was comforting for me just to know he was there. I wanted to sleep too. Sleep promised peace and escape from the relentless pain, but I was terrified that I wouldn't wake up. I really felt like this was it, and it annoyed me. What a way to go. This is not how it should happen, on a hospital trolley, in a dimly lit room, in agony. Part of me could have given up there and then, but another part was fighting back. I battled to keep my eyes open. If I had to die, I would much rather it be whilst I was doing something exciting; paragliding over the Alps would have been ideal. Not like this. It couldn't be like this. No.

It was about 1:30 a.m. when the doctor appeared with the CT results. "You have a bleed in your brain," she said, in the customary matter-of-fact manner. "There is a haemorrhage, but we're not sure whether it is inside or outside of your tumour. We don't have the facilities to deal with this here, so as soon as you are stable, we will be transferring you under blue lights to Walton Hospital, as that is the nearest neurological centre." I was told I was nil-by-mouth, and I couldn't even have a mouthful of water. Neil and I looked at each other. Damn, this really was getting too serious now.

"Can we go to Salford?" Neil asked, as that's where I was being treated.

"She's not stable enough to go that far. She must go to the nearest place, which is Walton." Chester to Walton is around

31 miles, and transfer would take approximately 40 minutes; Chester to Salford Royal is around 45 miles and could take approximately 50 minutes. When you can't chance a further 10 minutes, it really does underline the severity of the situation. Oh, lucky me!

My heart sank. I'd been worried that this would happen, and it was one of the main reasons why I didn't want to go to hospital in the first place. I think I was given steroids at this point and a few hours later, it was decided that I was stable enough to transfer to Walton, in Liverpool. As I was wheeled out of the emergency department, the nurses, who'd been taking care of me so well, wished me good luck. The paramedics then took over and conducted their own checks once I was in the ambulance, and when they were happy with my condition, we began our journey. Ambulances are surprisingly uncomfortable, especially when you're in severe pain. Every bump and jolt ripped through my skull. Could it get any worse? Yes, of course it could.

We arrived at Walton at about 5:00 a.m. It was already daylight, but ominous looking storm clouds were beginning to form in the hazy sky. I was wheeled into a ward of mostly elderly patients. Some were blissfully asleep, some were muttering incomprehensible things, and as I slowly made my way back from the bathroom, one lady asked if I could check under her bed, as she thought someone was hiding there; I've no idea how I managed it, but I crouched down, pretended to look, and reassured her. My records were updated, I was given another shot of steroids and fitted with some not-so-elegant compression stockings and colour-coded, pale blue, fall-risk socks; oh, hold me back on the glamour! Eventually, the pain started to recede, but not by much. It wasn't long until the on-call doctors came down to see me. They were surprised that I was being treated at Salford, as I lived within their catchment area. I felt quite awkward explaining that with Salford, I already had an operation date set in three weeks' time; with Walton, my initial appointment, if I'd chosen to accept it, was still over a month away. It's not always wise to upset the people who may be cracking your skull open at some point. I was told that the tumour had haemorrhaged and that it needed to come out. It was a medical emergency, a life-or-death situation, and surgery would either be later that day, or the following day at the very latest.

Part of me was relieved; perhaps this ordeal would be over sooner than anticipated, and that would surely be a bonus? But I also had my concerns. I had developed an excellent relationship with my surgeons at Salford. We had discussed the various risks associated with surgery, they knew my fears, and I trusted them implicitly to do everything possible to save my facial nerve. When I raised this point with the doctors now, the somewhat abrupt response was, "We'll discuss that when we go over the consent form." What? How would there be time to discuss anything at the consent form stage? Oh, no – I wasn't happy. For once, Doubt and I were in complete agreement. I told Neil I wouldn't be signing the consent form in that hospital and begged him to try to contact Salford, a task that wasn't easy in the early hours of a Sunday morning. Whilst the nurse was monitoring me, Neil disappeared off down the corridor to call Salford and email my consultant.

Have I told you how amazing my husband is? Somehow, and I still don't know how, he got through to the right people, and they responded. I could hear a phone call at a desk outside the ward, where I'm quite sure Professor Lloyd and Salford Royal were both mentioned. Minutes later, the consultant returned, explaining that Salford Royal had requested that as soon as my condition was stable, I was to be transferred to them. The relief was incredible, but I put on my poker face to conceal my pleasure at this development. It was about another half an hour before three paramedics arrived with another trolley to wheel me into an ambulance.

"Don't get up!" the doctor insisted as I was about to sit up and move myself onto it. He stopped me in my tracks and made me lie back down. He explained that Salford had insisted I wasn't to lift my head more than 30 degrees upright. Awkwardly, and with the help of Neil and the paramedics, I slid myself across the bed and onto the trolley. Once the paperwork was signed and my vital signs checked once again, we were back on the motorway, this time heading to Salford Royal, Manchester.

The journey was relatively quick, and when we arrived we were greeted at the door by the on-call neurosurgeon. I think his name was Alex. He was extremely reassuring, and we realised that we had him to thank for coordinating the transfer from Walton; it sounded almost like a prison break! He explained in more detail what had happened; the tumour had haemorrhaged and it was this that had caused the excruciating pain. It now appeared to have been brought under control by the high doses of steroids. Alex told us that whilst my consultant, Scott Rutherford, wasn't aware of my admission, he would be informed of the situation first thing the following morning and would no doubt come to see me. I was to be admitted for observation and for pain management; there would be no rush to discharge me and I could remain there as long as I felt I needed to.

True to Alex's word, Scott came to visit me the following morning, greeting me with, "What a pleasant, but unwanted surprise!" He explained that whilst it was very rare for tumours like mine to haemorrhage, it was not unheard of and it was documented. He explained that he didn't want to operate immediately, as he considered that the inflammation and damage caused by the bleeding would complicate surgery and increase the risks associated with it. I understood, but in a way, I was a little disappointed; I'd hoped that this would bring my surgery forward, a step closer to the end of this horrific journey. I continued to be closely monitored, and was discharged a few days later with a course of steroids to help everything settle down.

I really can't praise Salford Royal enough. My treatment was nothing short of outstanding. Everyone, and I do mean everyone, from the cleaners and porters, to housekeeping, to the nurses and the consultants, were amazing. Each and every one of them made time to talk to me, they spoke to me as though I was a normal human being and they checked not only that I was ok, but my family too. It was a reassuring and confidence-building 'dry run'. I cannot begin to explain how very grateful I was.

It was a huge relief to be home, but also the start of the longest three weeks of my life. It wasn't long before I was back in bed, and if I made any movement at all, I was throwing up. If I thought I'd been bad before, it was nothing compared to this. I was in almost daily contact with my specialist skull base surgery team who were checking up on me, just in case I needed urgent treatment, as I lived some distance away and the travel time needed to be factored in.

By the end of the first week, I was really beginning to think that I couldn't cope any longer. Eating was a huge challenge, because nothing appealed to me. Besides, I knew that my chances of hanging on to the food were slim, and the novelty of being sick had worn off long ago. I could just about walk to the next room, as long as I could cling on to furniture and use the walls for support, but my legs shook and I was frightened not only of falling, but not being able to get up if I did. There is nothing worse than the feeling of being horrendously drunk, without any of the enjoyment. Doubt was my almost constant companion, chatty little soul that he was, casting random dark thoughts in my direction, with a smirk. The thought I might die during surgery was a frequent one, as was the one where I might be better off dead, not only for myself, but for my family too; I was only existing and struggling to do that. I worried about my facial nerve; I wasn't vain, but I really did want to maintain the normality of a symmetrical, working face. The words hearing loss, loss of balance, facial paralysis, difficulty swallowing, tinnitus, double vision, headaches, fatigue, meningitis continued to roll through my thoughts as if on a loop, not exactly the catchy chorus that it might have been. Doubt stoked the feelings of anger, resentment and frustration; I had always looked after myself, eaten the right things and taken exercise, but why had I bothered, if I was just going to end up like this? Why hadn't I just become the dough-nut queen and enjoyed it? In secret, I wrote letters to Neil and my family, apologising for putting them all through this ordeal and telling them how much I loved them, just in case I didn't make it. I kept receiving those messages from well-meaning friends and family saying, "You'll beat this", "Stay strong" and "Keep fighting". The reality of brain tumours and many other serious illnesses, though, is very different. It just doesn't work like that. I always thought I was a fighter, but when you don't have the strength to stand long enough to shower, fighting is out of the question. These supposedly encouraging comments were far from helpful; they just add another burden on people who are already incredibly sick and very scared.

Once again, in my moment of need, I received a message from my Navy friends. They were a constant source of knowledge and support, whenever it came to my latest crazy challenge, and in some respects, this was no different, other than it wasn't my choice. People I'd spoken to about my situation had told me that I would get used to my 'new normal'. I didn't want a new normal. I liked my old normal and I wanted to keep hold of that. I had a full-on rant; why had I bothered making the effort to train and to keep fit? It hadn't been worth it, and it certainly hadn't got me very far.

They listened, they gave me time to vent and then they replied. In their own typical fashion, their messages were short and sweet.

"Think again," was their thought-provoking response. They were right. Putting all of that hard work in had placed me in a stronger position than most to deal with this. I had given myself an undeniable advantage and the best possible chance. Whilst it didn't seem that way right now, it would help me with my recovery. They told me I had to be both positive and aggressive to deal with what lay ahead. We unravelled my concerns, and I came to realise that my biggest worries were the unknowns, along with not wanting to give someone else the control over my outcome. I had to let go of any control and trust my surgeons, which was bizarre, as I did trust them, but I needed to trust them on a deeper level; was just inside my skull deep enough?

"This is what they do," they told me. I needed to trust them to do their job, and I did, but there was still a 'but' hanging in the air. It's a bit like when you trust a pilot to fly the plane you're travelling in. Easy to say in theory, but when it's your brain they're dealing with, well that's a whole different ball game.

I had to stop counting down the days to what I thought was the end, and now consider it as day one of a new beginning. From that day I would know exactly what I'd be dealing with, and once I knew that, I could start to work on my recovery. It sounded like an ideal solution; the problem was that I didn't know how to do it. They taught me how to break things down into small, manageable pieces. I had to stop looking at the big picture because that was terrifying and self-destructive. It was essential to focus on whatever was immediately in front of me, to take life one day at a time, one hour at a time, or even one minute at a time if necessary. Complete that one small task, then move onto the next thing. They told me I needed to be patient with my recovery too; this was major brain surgery and it was going to take a whole lot of time, probably more than my wildest estimate, to recover. They told me of people they served with who'd had severe head injuries and the timescales involved. This would be normal, to be expected, and even though I wouldn't like it, I needed to be prepared for it.

Many people would tell me what I wanted to hear, which I completely understand and probably would have done myself, but these individuals, well they always say it as it is. For me, this is perfect and I really admire their blunt honesty. Everything is either black or white; there are no grey areas. As they said, grey areas leave room for doubt and questions; in their job, they have no room for that. The result would be catastrophic. Whilst this is very applicable to anyone in their line of work, it can also be relevant to everyday life for the rest of us. How many times do we overcomplicate things with ifs, buts and maybes? Similarly, how often do we use words such as wish, could, might and maybe, without realising just how negative those words can be? Ditch them and instead say I can and I will, and really mean it. Do something that brings you closer to fulfilling your goal every single day. It doesn't have to be much, just keep moving forward.

For me, this conversation was a game-changer, as all the pieces fell into place. In fact, when I look back, I'd go so far as to say it was life changing. The first thing I did was change the countdown timer I'd set on my phone from 'Days left' to 'Days until I get my life back'. A positive action. Doubt was most grumpy over the whole thing.

CHAPTER 3

12th May 2018. D-day. I had been so exhausted these last few weeks that despite the seriousness of the situation, I think my brain had taken pity on me and allowed me to sleep, and not only sleep but to sleep well. Neil woke me at 5:00 a.m. when the alarm went off; he didn't say anything, but I don't think he'd been as lucky as me on the sleep front. I had been nil-by-mouth since midnight and was only allowed fluids until 6:00 a.m., due to the anaesthetic.

The drive to Manchester was remarkably lovely. It was a clear, bright morning, the start of another warm, sunny day. In another time, another place, I might have been preparing to go hiking in the mountains. Mist had settled over the fields, sparkling with dew and looking almost magical. Surprisingly, a sense of calm had settled over me, and almost optimism; I had finally accepted all my fears and misgivings and realised that the entire situation was out of my hands. I had no choice but to let others get on and do their job; to trust their tremendous skills. The only thing I could do was to build upon the foundations of their work and ensure the best possible recovery for myself.

The previous week had been difficult in more ways than I could have imagined, with Doubt constantly by my side. Just the previous day, I'd been invited to a hospital appointment and told by the happy, smiley doctor who'd previously given me my brain tumour diagnosis that abnormalities on my lung X-rays and CT scan would need further investigation, as there was a possibility that this could be lymphoma. He asked when I would be available for these investigations to take place, to which I replied, "I'm having brain surgery tomorrow." There was a pause before he replied, telling me that I would need to have biopsies taken as soon as it was physically possible. Well, wasn't that just something else to look forward to? So we left the hospital, not only with thoughts of my impending surgery but uncertain of what the future would hold beyond that. What new battle did we now potentially face? Again, I felt numb to my situation, almost detached from it I suppose. This seemed to be my way of coping with everything, if you can call it coping. Those things I had no control of were being shut away in the back of my mind, whilst I focussed on the immediate future.

I had spent days combing the internet for the tiniest glimmers of hope that everything would be ok. There were very few glimmers to be had. Time after time, I found stories of facial paralysis that left people deeply upset and distressed, the need for nerve grafts, the inability to walk unaided, those unable to return to their career, or any sort of work, the ones that didn't make it... My heart went out to each one of them. It was hard, if not impossible, to find anything positive; the internet appears to thrive on tales of death, destruction and despair. Any of those things could happen to me. All of those things could happen to me. Doubt did somersaults of pure joy.

For weeks it felt as though half of my head was being invaded, made worse by the fact that the other half felt relatively normal, so I could compare and contrast with ease. It was utterly relentless; a heavy, sickening fog that made even the simplest of tasks challenging beyond belief. I struggled with the term 'new normal'; I didn't want that to be me. I was beyond exhausted, but somewhere, deep inside me, the first flickers of the flames to get back out there and fight were starting to stir. If there were any chance at all, even 0.1%, of retaining me, I was determined to do it. If this acoustic neuroma and its after-effects wanted a battle, I was going to give it a war.

At that hour, the hospital car park was almost empty; on the plus side, it was easy to park, which is always a bonus. In direct contrast to the bright sunshine of outside, we were directed through endless long, dimly lit corridors until we reached the surgical admissions department. It was just minutes before we were called through to the ward. My stomach turned somersaults. This really was the point of no return. I was the centre of attention as nurses came along and took MRSA (Methicillin-resistant Staphylococcus aureus) swabs and blood and urine samples, and checked my blood pressure, pulse and temperature, all of which were recorded. There was even a pregnancy test, which was undoubtedly the biggest waste of time and money, but good for comedy value, if nothing else. Doubt casually pointed out that any of these had the potential to stop the surgery. Thanks for that; I was fully aware of the situation. Just when I thought things couldn't get any better, I was handed the hospital gowns, surgical stockings and paper pants. There's nothing quite like looking your very best for the occasion. The waiting began.

Scott had previously reassured me that on the day I wouldn't be left waiting for long, and he was right. It was only half an hour, but it's amazing how far time can stretch. Neil and I sat together, trying to pretend that everything was ok, but it was just about as far from ok as it was possible to be. I listened to the lady in the next bed talking about her gall bladder operation. If only. Who would have thought that operation envy was a thing?

I was visited by my team, firstly Joe Sebastian, my anaesthetist, who talked me through what would happen when I got to the operating theatre. That didn't sound too bad, in the grand scheme of things. Scott Rutherford and Simon Lloyd were next up, with the consent form. Scott explained to Neil that surgery could take 12 hours or more and that he was not to worry if it did; picking the tumour away from the nerves was delicate and time-consuming work, and it didn't mean that anything had gone wrong. I could see Neil nodding, grateful for anything that added to his 'knowledge is power' coping mechanism. I wondered if the gall bladder lady was listening.

Simon began to read through the consent form and the list of possible side effects of the surgery; I knew that list as well as my name. Once he was about halfway through, he looked at me and said, "You really don't want me to go through all of this again, do you?"

"Just let me get back to the mountains and try not to mess my face up," was my reply. Simon started to amend the form to show that I was giving consent for additional surgery; an abdominal fat harvest and also a nerve graft, if it was necessary. My surgery involved the removal of a section of my skull and the resulting hole would be filled with my abdominal fat; good luck finding any of that after the last few months. The nerve graft would be necessary if my facial nerve were compromised; they would attempt to give me some of the function back by replacing the nerve. The reality of seeing that in black and white was incredibly hard. With a shaking hand and a lump in my throat, I signed my name as best I could. Simon drew an arrow on the left side of my neck and they left to finish preparing the theatre. It was really happening.

The next 15 minutes were rather tearful ones before the porter arrived with the trolley. I tried to hold back the tears, as I said "See you later," to Neil.

His reply of "I love you" broke me. I realised that it was the last time my left ear would hear those most precious words if indeed I ever heard them again.

Unstoppable tears rolled down my cheeks, as I was pushed away from Neil and along the ward; even now, I can't bear to think of how Neil must have felt. The porter, sensing my distress, did his very best to distract me. He was a tall man, with a strong Mancunian accent and a vast array of conversation topics. I wish I had known his name, as not only was he brilliant at his job, but he displayed incredible kindness too; he deserves to be on the thank you list. It took about 10 minutes to reach the theatre; does anyone appreciate how fit porters must be? The miles they must walk? The porter tried a football conversation, which was a non-starter, as I'm not a fan, and then he tried holidays. Perfect. We chatted about my recent trip to the Alps, how breathtakingly beautiful the scenery was, how crisp the air felt, and how I loved walking. Yes, I loved walking. With impeccable timing, Doubt appeared, and cheerfully asked, "What if you can never do that again?" Oh, don't you worry, if there is any way, and I do mean any, I will be back out there, and out there sooner rather than later.

Moments later, we arrived at the operating theatre; I'm not sure what I expected, but it wasn't this. From the outside, it looked like a heavy, industrial fridge door, and when it opened it could have been just that. I was wheeled into a small room that led into the main theatre. Joe was waiting there, with his assistant, and they quickly got to work sticking pads to my chest, inserting cannulas, and putting blood pressure monitors on. Oh, how I wanted to turn tail and run. Every fibre of me wanted to run, although the reality would have been a bit of a stagger and possibly an unsophisticated slump onto the spotlessly clean floor. I could feel my pulse beginning to race as they did their best to make me feel at ease, and more importantly, confident in their abilities. I think by this point, especially after the haemorrhage, everyone knew that I really had very little left to give. I was given oxygen through a mask, whilst the anaesthetic was administered. I felt my eyelids becoming heavy, as the surprisingly cold liquid snaked up my arm. In seconds I was out of it.

I woke quite suddenly, in a small room, with two nurses by my side. For a moment, I didn't know where I was and felt very disorientated, and then I remembered; to be honest, the nurses were a bit of a clue. I felt surprisingly wide awake, as a wave of relief washed over me; I'd had my surgery, and not only that, I'd survived. That was one in the eye for Doubt, for sure.

I assessed myself, as you do, just to make sure that everything was present and correct. Unsurprisingly, my head didn't feel right; the only way to describe it was as though it was being squashed, and as it goes, it was pretty uncomfortable. Ah, yes, that would be the compression bandage I'd been told about, to reduce the risk of leakage. Leakage. Have you noticed that nothing good is ever associated with the word 'leakage'? I knew that the compression bandage would have to remain in place for a few days, so I'd better get used to that one. My throat felt dry and sore, most likely from tubes being stuck down there whilst I was asleep. I had cannulas everywhere and was hooked up to drips and all sorts of machinery, but that was to be expected and a good thing. OK, I could live with that. My vision was rubbish, but no glasses when you need them will do that, so I asked the nurse to my left if she could pass them to me. Speaking felt a little different and I'm sure I slurred my words, as you do when you've had one or two too many. She reached over to get them, so that was another tick, as at least I could still talk and be understood. Things were going well. The nurse placed the glasses on my head, as best she could, given the dressings; it was a struggle.

"Oh, for heaven's sake", I thought. "What have they been doing with them?" They were filthy and I couldn't see! Feeling as though I were a nuisance, I asked if she could just give the lenses a quick wipe for me. There was a pause before she calmly told me that they were clean. Rubbish, they must have had something smeared all over them, and if she couldn't see that… oh. It wasn't the glasses, it was me. I couldn't see. Well, I could, but it was as though I was looking through thick fog. Oh, hello Panic, I knew you wouldn't be far away.

Still wearing scrubs, Scott appeared from behind a curtain at the end of my bed; I could just about make him out.

"It went really, really well Sara," he said. "It took us far less time than we thought it would, and to be honest, after the haemorrhage, we were concerned about what we would find once we opened up. We managed to remove all of it." He added that the tumour came away from the nerves considerably well, although they had to be manipulated quite a bit. I had a grade 3 facial palsy, but he reassured me that my facial nerve was functioning when they closed up and he was confident that any paralysis would resolve over time. He added that he would call Neil straight away and let him know I was out of theatre.

I thanked him. I knew that if necessary a sliver of tumour might be left behind, if it was felt that removing it would compromise my facial nerve. I knew this, and had come to terms with this and the prospect of radiation treatment for any regrowth, should it be necessary, but I hadn't realised just how relieved I would be to hear that they removed 100% of it. I felt like a huge weight had been lifted. I continued with my assessment. I couldn't see; now that was a real concern, as I'd quit a reasonably secure job to be a photographer, and being able to see was kind of essential for that. What if that was permanent? Park that thought for now, as at the moment there was nothing I could do about it. My hearing didn't bother me at that point – my head was covered in bandage anyway, and everything was muffled. My face, well I couldn't feel half of it, and that was weird. From my forehead to below my chin was totally numb, with no sensation at all. Even the inside of my mouth was numb. I could have drawn a line right down the centre of my tongue; on the right side it felt normal, on the left I couldn't feel a thing. Talking really is somewhat awkward when you can't feel your tongue and half your mouth. It was so completely numb that I reckon I could have had root canal surgery without anaesthetic. Could I live with it? Probably. The absolute best thing though, was that the horrible, horrible feeling in my head, that I'd lived with for months, was practically gone.

Then I was sick. Used to seeing the effects of this kind of surgery, as if by magic, the nurse deftly thrust a bowl right in front of me. As I bent forward to throw up, I felt a searing, stabbing pain in my stomach; oh, yes – that would be the site of the fat harvest; they found some then. As an extra layer of unexpected delight, there was a drain inserted into my stomach wound, and each time I moved it dug in, with extremely painful consequences. Marvellous.

It took about half an hour for me to stop vomiting, and I wondered if they'd thought of using a stomach drain as the ultimate deterrent. A third nurse appeared, and they moved me up to the neuro high-dependency unit, where I had a room to myself. There is something quite sobering when you realise that one of your entourage is carrying an automated electrical defibrillator. I hoped that this was standard procedure and they didn't expect me to croak en route, but, when you think about it, I had been through a lot and perhaps there was a certain severity to my situation.

The room was large; the bed was anchored into place, with my back against the windows. I was hooked up to monitors that were recording my heart rate, blood pressure, respiration, and oxygen saturation levels. I had a catheter and the stomach drain, saline drips and other bags of medication feeding directly into my bloodstream. Not exactly dignified, but essential. I looked like a mini power station with all the cables hanging from my poor battered and bruised body.

Moments later, I heard my mum and Neil in the corridor and they were shown into my room. I tried to gauge how I looked from their reactions, but my eyesight wasn't up to it.

"How are you feeling?" Neil asked. As soon as I heard his voice, the relief that I'd made it this far turned into tears, and all I could say was "Do I look like a freak?"

"Of course you don't!" he replied, trying his best to comfort me, but unable to find anywhere that looked safe to touch. He even took photos to help convince me. OK, so, I didn't look like a complete freak, but I certainly looked a mess; I looked like someone who had been through many hours of brain surgery. It was at this time that I realised my left eye wasn't working properly. When I cried, there were no tears. I suppose it wasn't worth crying if I could only half cry. Although they couldn't stay for long, my mum and Neil chatted away, whilst I fought to keep my eyes open. The sense of relief was palpable for all of us. The nurse continually checked that everything was as it should be. By now, I had little energy to talk; with half of my mouth and tongue completely numb, and being unable to swallow properly, speaking was difficult. I had read about this as a potential problem and desperately hoped that along with my face and my vision, this issue would resolve itself in time, although sooner rather than later would have been very good indeed.

I was woken every 30 minutes for a neurological check, which is a way of assessing that everything is as it should be. I had to push and pull against the nurses' hands with my hands and feet, grip their fingers, lift my arms, smile and open and close my eyes as physical checks. I was asked my name, what day it was and which hospital I was in, to monitor for any confusion. Any signs of weakness could indicate a stroke or other injury to my brain. All the other usual observations were done too: heart rate, respiratory rate, blood pressure and temperature. I'd never felt so popular.

Eventually, I managed to fall asleep, until I was again woken for my observations. As I opened my eyes, the strangest thing happened; not only was my vision rubbish, but everything appeared to be tilted on its side. The door at the end of my bed was sloping to the right, at a 45-degree angle. Surely not. Was I dreaming? I blinked a few times, and it righted itself. I tried to stay awake in case it happened again, but the stress of the day and the cocktail of medication I'd been given were all too much, and once I'd finished vomiting (that drain!) I drifted off once again.

I woke with a start, and as I opened my eyes, everything appeared to be tipped on its side again. Not satisfied with the 45 degrees of last time, it was now 90 degrees. Blinking didn't clear it. It was the weirdest sensation and I felt as though I was going to fall out of bed, although somewhere deep inside, logic was telling me that it wasn't possible. I gripped the rail with one hand, and frantically pressed the buzzer with the other, not realising that the nurse was stationed in my room at the time. Trying to control the panic, I explained what was happening; not only could I not see properly through one eye, but everything I could see was now on its side. My vision was so badly distorted that I could see the clock directly above the door, and I could also see a second clock and second door, about 2 m across the room, which I knew for a fact were not there; both were on their side too. The wash hand basin was no longer on the wall, but on the floor, and people coming into my room appeared to be walking on the walls. It was disorientating and terrifying. It certainly hadn't been on the list of possible side effects and I'd seen no mention of this on the internet. The nystagmus had also worsened, with my left eye seemingly jumping around uncontrollably as I tried to focus on the nurse. Trust me to be different.

The nurse was reassuring and explained that these things can sometimes happen and I shouldn't worry, but she would mention it to the charge nurse. A short time later, the charge nurse came in to see me. She agreed with the nurse and also said not to worry but she would mention it to the on-call neurosurgeons, who were on duty that particular night. As I lay there, with my world tipped on its side, I noticed that the sippy cup that I'd been drinking water from was also on its side, appearing to defy gravity. What was really strange, however, was that the water line was straight, as it would have been if it had been the right way up. I tried to rationalise my situation; my world wasn't tipped over on its side, it was just my perception of it at the time. I focussed on a point in the room – for example, the footboard at the end of my bed – and tried to see it as it should be, as in the right way up. Have you ever been on a haunted house fairground ride, where the floors are uneven and there are mirrors that distort everything, so you are completely disorientated? It was very similar to that, only it wasn't going to be over in three minutes and there was no exit sign. I was exhausted and terrified; what if I needed further surgery to correct this? Doubt nodded in agreement; of course, it was possible. I fought desperately to stay awake. I don't think I've ever felt so alone or scared.

It must have been a couple of hours later that the on-call neuro came to see me. Again, he did his best to reassure me that this can occasionally happen and I shouldn't worry. My brain and nerves had been manipulated quite a bit to get to and to remove the tumour, which meant that everything was a little angry and inflamed. I knew the feeling.

"Can I have a quick word outside?" he asked the nurse who was assigned to me. As they left my room, I heard him say that they wouldn't worry too much about this, at least for the first 48 hours, but to keep a close eye on me. Hmmm… not as common as everyone was making out then. Salford Royal… your walls are thinner than you think. I couldn't really say what I felt at that time other than absolute fear and panic. For those few hours, I was terrified that this is what the rest of my life would be like. Doubt stoked the fears. The sickness increased and I felt as though I was choking as I struggled to swallow. Each time I threw up, I had a sharp pain in my stomach from the drain. Eventually, I lost my battle to stay awake and despite being woken every 30 minutes, I slept the rest of the night. Hand on heart, I think that was quite possibly the worst and most frightening night of my life.

I was woken by a different nurse the following morning. She was bubbly and chatted away to me as I tried to fully wake myself up and focus. I think she said she was from the Philippines; I can't remember her name, but along with so many others, she needs to be on the thank you list. She tried to persuade me to have a cup of tea, but I was still being sick; I'd not had a drink of tea or coffee for weeks, as my taste buds were so messed up. Nothing tasted as it should do; if I drank cola, on the right side of my tongue it tasted normal, but on the left side, it was tasteless, just like soda water. So, I stuck to water. Foods were either tasteless or metallic. Thankfully, my world had started to right itself ever so slightly, so as the nurse helped me to wash, I remained focused on the end of my bed, willing myself to see the world correctly again.

Having heard I'd had a difficult night, I had a visitor: one of my surgeons, Simon Lloyd. He too did his best to reassure me that there was nothing to worry about, but it didn't work this time; I'm sorry, but I knew about the 48-hour thing, and that when a doctor tells a nurse to keep an eye on you when you're already in a neuro high-dependency ward, things are potentially a little bit precarious. Simon explained that once they'd got into my head, they'd found far more hairs in my inner ear than they were expecting; the gentamicin should have destroyed these, but the injections hadn't been as effective as they hoped. Ideally, I'd needed one or two more for it to have been completely effective, but I'd run out of time. He reconfirmed that there had been a lot of manipulation of the nerves and everything would be inflamed. Foiled by hairy ears; who would have thought it?

"Don't look so terrified!" he said in his usual calm, reassuring way, as he turned to leave.

"Easy for you to say," I thought to myself, feeling surprisingly petulant. I was terrified. I'd tried so hard to put a brave face on it, but this was my life; this was potentially how the rest of my life would be and there wasn't a workaround for it. Doubt nodded in complete agreement.

People came and went, checking everything. It appeared that I was doing well, apart from the vomiting and the double vision.

My heart rate and blood pressure were back down to more normal levels, no doubt due to the reduction of the pressure on my brainstem. As the day went on, the major issues I'd had with my vision settled down ever so slightly, but I was scared of falling asleep, in case it all went wrong again. In the day, Neil and my mum came to see me, and in the evening, it was my dad and my brother; I ended up in that strange situation where although I craved the company, and the reassurance of familiar people, I couldn't cope with it; I was struggling with feeling so unlike my normal self and trying to hide it. Rather than all of the unknowns, I just wanted to know exactly what I was dealing with.

Due to the issues I'd experienced, I spent an additional night on the high-dependency unit. I remember lying there, wanting, and needing, to sleep but feeling too scared to do so. There were problems for the poor man in the next room to mine. I could hear the staff trying to wake him, as he had become unresponsive; the hurried footsteps, the sense of urgency, the voices pitched at a level that was difficult to ignore, and the rattle of equipment. Even listening to it felt like an intrusion; I tried to block everything out. Doubt wouldn't let me; he reminded me of how easily that could have been me. Somewhere nearby, another man was crying out in pain.

The following morning brought the physio team to my side. I was on anticoagulants (blood thinners) and wearing inflatable sleeves around my lower legs, that inflated and deflated to maintain my circulation, but there was still a concern that I could develop blood clots. The physios were tasked with trying to get me moving as soon as possible. A chair was brought into my room and placed roughly a metre away. The two physios helped me to sit up and moved all of the drips and monitors, unhooking the drain and catheter. Slowly, they sat me upright on the side of the bed, before lowering it, so my feet could touch the floor and I could put them in slippers. The physios positioned themselves with one on either side of me and helped me to stand.

Oh boy, was that unexpected. Just standing felt completely alien to me. I was rooted to the spot, my eyes transfixed on the chair in front of me, which was so close, I think I could have reached out and touched it. "OK," said one of the physios, reassuringly, "We're just going to walk to the chair and you can sit in it for a while."

"Easy," I thought to myself, as I went to take a step. I focused on the wall ahead of me and tried to move my leg. Not so easy, my leg didn't move. It was the same as the difficulty with my handwriting; my brain knew what my legs needed to do, and was sending the usual instructions, but my legs were not receiving them. It felt as though I was wearing lead weights on my feet. Just six months ago, I was running half marathons, and now, a metre was practically out of reach. I didn't dare to move my head in case I was sick; the thought of two vomit-splattered physios was not a happy one. I was scared of wobbling, as I knew I had no reactions to correct it. After about 15 minutes of shuffle, rest, shuffle, rest, and giving it everything I'd got, I made it. I don't think I've ever been so glad to see a blue armchair in my life. Half marathons took far less effort than that.

All my tubes and bags were hung back up, and I sank back into that armchair, my new best friend. I was completely exhausted, to the point where I was trembling. That was the moment I realised the enormity of what lay ahead; I hadn't been far wrong when I'd thought of it as a war. I wanted to cry, but I didn't have the energy to, and besides, I couldn't even do that properly.

Later that evening, it was considered that I'd made sufficient progress to be transferred into a room on the neuro ward. Everything that Neil had brought in for me was packed up, and I was wheeled up to the ward; a moment that was marred, as I began to be sick again. I hadn't eaten for days now, and my stomach was hurting; there was nothing to throw up, other than the occasional sips of water that I'd managed to keep down for a while, at least. I'd reached the point of being scared of being sick, in case I dislodged the drain or the lump of fat in my skull, which with the support of a few stitches and a tight bandage was holding my brain in place. Doubt and I had run through the list of potential setbacks on more than one occasion; I didn't want any of them.

The room was almost identical to the one I'd been in a few weeks earlier. My mum had brought along some get well cards that people had sent, and some gorgeous flowers, which she organised in a pretty display on top of my bedside locker. I was still hooked up to all sorts of paraphernalia, and whilst it was still an achievement to be away from the high-dependency unit, I was nowhere near where I wanted to be. I finally felt up to checking my phone; Neil had brought it in for me each day, but until now I'd sent it straight back home. As I turned it on, the first message to pop up was from my friends in the Navy, hoping they weren't too late to wish me luck with my op. It had been sent the day after my surgery (typical Navy timing), and it meant everything. I replied, and moments later, so did they.

"We're so proud of you… now show us what you're made of, and show the docs what a Navy recovery is like. Send us pics of your recovery, we want to be there with you!" How's that for motivation?

Naively, I'd thought I would be going home on Wednesday, but when Wednesday morning arrived, I still hadn't eaten and there were concerns about my blood sugar levels dropping. The dressing on my head was removed, which was instant relief, if a short-lived one; my ear expanded out of the side of my head, raising concerns that I had developed a CSF leak (leaking cerebrospinal fluid, the liquid that surrounds your spine and brain), which can be serious. My catheter was removed, allowing me some extra freedom – not that I was up to venturing very far.

Each day, the physio came to see me; as lovely as he was, I dreaded his visits. With an eye patch in place, to help with the double vision and nystagmus, I must have looked like an inebriated pirate, wobbling around all over the place after a night on the grog; all I needed was the beard and the parrot to complete the look. He would take me out of my room to walk up and down the corridor, holding tightly onto the handrail; not quite the change of scenery that I craved. He made the suggestion that when I was discharged, it would be a good idea for me to have a walking frame. There was a pause before he added that he could see from the expression on my face I wasn't too keen on that idea. Absolutely right I wasn't. He explained that before I could be discharged, I would need to pass the 'stair test', to ensure that I could manage the stairs. The following day, I made him take me to the stairs to practise. He asked which side the bannister rail was on at home and I said the right; the truth was that we didn't have one. Once again, I found myself doing something that felt as though I'd never done it before, but I was ready for it. I pushed every other thought from my mind and concentrated on the 'lift, forward, down'; my life may not have depended on it, but my freedom certainly did. Each step was calculated and felt rather precarious. It was a very tentative turn that I made at the top and a cautious descent. I passed the test. Although I was delighted with this, as it was quite an achievement, it didn't take long for Doubt to appear, "Not exactly a mountain, though, is it?" Sadly, I couldn't argue with him.

I had been told to stay in bed and call for assistance if I needed to go to the bathroom, which was near the end of my bed and just a couple of metres away. I had been drinking and keeping down so little, the toilet wasn't an issue anyway, right up to the time when it was, so I rang the bell and I waited. I hated being so dependent on others for the everyday things that the majority of us take for granted, especially as everyone was so busy. It wasn't long until I needed to go again; I looked at the door to my room, closed as always. I could, if I was very careful, try and get there myself. No one would ever know.

I did a quick risk assessment. If I stood up from the chair alongside my bed and held on to the small, wheeled table, you know, the ones you find alongside hospital beds, I could use that as a handrail to get to the end of the bed. From the end of the bed, I'd be able to reach the bathroom door handle. Once I had opened the door, there was a rail on the inside of it and from there I could use the wash hand basin to help me get to the toilet. I went for it. Every section was a challenge all of its own, and as I completed each one, I congratulated myself accordingly. After the event, I stood up, washed my hands, and shuffled back towards the door, revelling in my moment of triumph. Just as I opened the door, the nurse walked into my room. The expression on her face said everything; to say she wasn't impressed was a bit of an understatement!

The following afternoon, I had visitors. Lots of visitors. Neil, my parents, and Neil's cousin Sue, who worked at Salford as a radiographer. Sue had been a great companion during my time on the high-dependency unit, popping in during her breaks and keeping me supplied with magazines and sweets. Soon after, my aunt and uncle arrived. It was quite a party, with everyone enjoying the opportunity to catch up. Except me. With my bandages removed, and this being my first exposure to a considerable level of noise, I felt totally out of my depth and unable to cope. The voices all merged into a cacophony of sound; I just couldn't focus on what one person was saying, and the fact that half the conversation was in Spanish made things even worse. As I was told numerous times how lucky I was, and how it was all over now and I could get back to normal, I struggled to hold back the tears from the one eye that still worked. I prayed for them to go, and when the door finally closed behind them, I fell apart. For years, I had worked in special needs education. Ironically, just before I resigned I had been working with a profoundly deaf child. I had attended all the deaf awareness courses, studied everything I could to do with sensory deficits, and even learnt some BSL

(British Sign Language) to help him access the curriculum. But nothing, nothing, can prepare you for waking up and finding yourself in this very different world.

It wasn't long after that I was assessed by occupational health, with a view to going home. I had to show that I could get to the bathroom independently, wash, clean my teeth, get dressed, and so on; all of the basics, really. A part of me felt this was totally irrelevant to me and a waste of everyone's time, but as I stood there, wobbling in front of the mirror, trying to put toothpaste on my toothbrush without falling against the wall, I had a bit of a rethink; I realised how necessary this was. I also realised how far I still had to go for just the basics to be comfortable, never mind the targets I had planned. Daunted? Who me? Most definitely, and I didn't need Doubt for that.

CHAPTER 4

Six days after my surgery, I left the hospital. I was dosed up on anti-sickness medication, wearing an eye patch and armed with a bag of pills, including laxatives. No one tells you about that fun part! I was determined not to use a walking frame unless I had absolutely no choice in the matter; luck was on my side for once, and thankfully I could get by without.

At the time of my diagnosis, I did what everyone does, and immersed myself in the internet, looking for hope. As previously mentioned, there was very little in the way of positivity, and the online support groups didn't do much to alleviate my worries. Neil did his best to convince me that for every negative comment online, there could well be 10 positive outcomes, where people had recovered and moved on in life. I now think there's some truth in that. Someone else pointed out that support groups often have people who are not coping very well, and will, therefore, be heavily weighted in that direction; I think there's some truth in that too.

With the best of intentions, many people told me that I would get used to the new normal. Every single time I heard that it filled me with frustration, anger and a sense of helplessness, which combined into a rage to the point where I felt physically sick. Little Miss Furious was a frequent visitor. I didn't want the new normal. In fact, I really regretted that I hadn't taken the time to like and appreciate myself properly, before the start of this nightmare. I have the utmost respect for every single person who has had their life decimated in some way, to the point where they can't achieve much or any of their previous normal, and yet they carve themselves a new path, with a grit and determination that few can appreciate. Yes, you can say that they had no choice, and in many ways that's true, but attitude is everything. Some sections of my normal were unaffected; my home, my family, some of my friends, but many areas I loved with all my heart were in jeopardy. I was determined that my new normal, if I had to have one, would be even better than the old one.

I work best when I have a target, a goal to be achieved, and I'd already put a few of those in place. My first target was the Race for Life in Chester, which I'd entered before my surgery. There was a lot of work to be done between now and then, but if I could make it, I was going to be there for sure. At that stage, crawling on my hands and knees was not out of the question.

I began to venture out, with caution, two weeks after my surgery. That summer, the weather was glorious and Britain basked in an unusual heatwave. Neil and I, together with our dog Hugo, ventured to the local cycleway and began our slow walk. The sun on my skin felt amazing, as did the warm, fresh air. I was wobbly at times and on several occasions swerved uncontrollably, generally into the biggest patch of stinging nettles I could find; honestly, they were like a magnet to me – see nettles, throw myself in there. I didn't care; any pain from the nettle stings was a reminder of just how good it was to be alive, to be doing something I enjoyed, and to be doing something that didn't involve hospitals. It was also interesting to note that Doubt didn't like the sunshine and wasn't keen on walking. I was making progress.

I had set myself the target of walking just a single kilometre, as a test distance, if you like. I had been apprehensive about going further than this, but as I reached the 500-metre mark and my intended return point, I did a quick assessment as to how I was getting on; I felt good. Really good. Could I carry on? I thought so. Should I carry on? Possibly not, but Neil was with me, we could stop at any time, and sometimes you just have to say, "What the hell..." We pressed on. With every step, I scoured the ground as best I could, for bumps, tree roots, and anything that might cause me to tumble, as at that point I had the rare skill of tripping on fresh air. My neck was aching with the unaccustomed posture of constantly looking down. We continued to the gate at the end of the path, turned around, and came back. I was wearing my fitness watch for the first time in ages and used it to check the distance we'd covered; 2.3 kilometres. Never did I think that I'd be so excited to see 2.3 kilometres! OK, compared to what I could do a few months ago, it was no big distance, but if you think about the effort it took to walk one metre to the blue armchair, roughly three weeks before, this was huge progress! Pass me the gold medal, someone! I was utterly elated, but a little thought was forming at the back of my mind. If I'd made this much progress already, what would I be capable of in a few weeks? Not that I was impatient or anything...

As soon as we got home, I sat down to excitedly relive every step, and promptly fell asleep; the payback for such a great morning. I had convinced myself that the fatigue wouldn't last and it was just what my body needed to do to achieve recovery. The visible scars were healing well, but inside my head was still an unknown quantity; I really needed to remember that.

The weeks that followed surgery were a mix of sitting around, doing little in the way of sudden movements or bending, and trying to achieve a few modified yoga poses that would challenge my remaining balance system. I spent a lot of time standing precariously on one leg with my eyes closed, trying desperately not to hold onto the chair that was there as my safety net! I think my family were used to me doing slightly crazy things, as no one said a word about it as I stood there, sometimes statue-still and sometimes with windmill arms.

One thing I was not prepared for was that all the stress and worries that I had before my surgery just seemed to morph into a different set of stress and worries after it; I didn't get the level of long-term relief that I was expecting, which was strange and disappointing. I found that when I was tired, my head would ache around the area of the wound; I would worry that I had developed a dreaded CSF leak and all the problems associated with it. I worried about everything; Neil going to work, the children being out and about, lack of money, and how I was going to cover my outgoings, any time something felt different with me – it was if my coping mechanisms were functioning at 5% capacity and it was frightening. I struggled with basic things; some of the blue internal stitches, which should have dissolved, were rejected by my body. I knew this could happen and it was nothing to worry about, but I didn't cope well with it. The stitches were forced out of my scalp; they were irritating and sore, and eventually, I pulled out a few of the ones that got stuck, using tweezers. These were the times that Doubt always seemed to be lurking, insisting that it was only a matter of time before there was a major setback and that everything I'd achieved so far would fall apart. I feared that he was right; how could he not be right?

It was around this point in time when I was invited along for a PIP (Personal Independence Payment) assessment. PIP is available to anyone over the age of 16, whether they're working or not, if they have a health condition or disability that has caused difficulty with daily living or getting around for the last 3 months and expect those difficulties to continue for at least a further 9 months. As far as I was concerned, I ticked every box. I woke after a particularly disturbed night, as Doubt had been very chatty and I'd been worrying about this assessment process; it was something totally new to me, at a time where I was struggling in general, and there was little information or

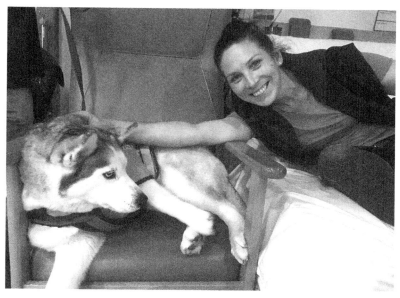

Meeting Ika, a Pets As Therapy dog, during my first admission to hospital following concerns raised by my GP, February 2018.

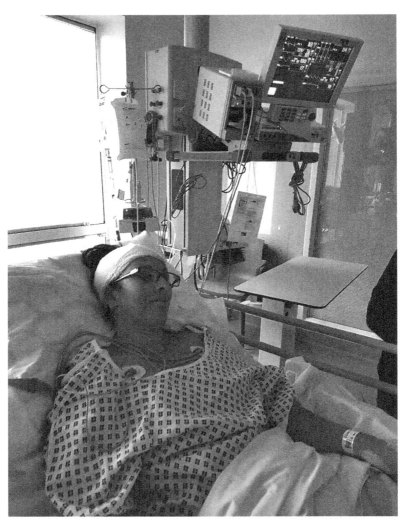

On HDU following surgery on 12th May 2018.

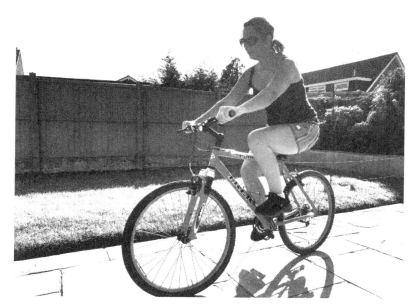

Learning to ride a bike again, 3 weeks after surgery.

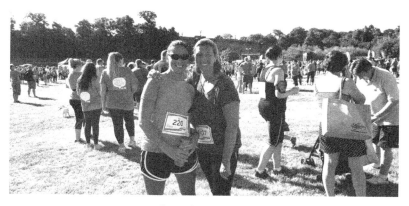

Chester Race for Life, 8 weeks after surgery.

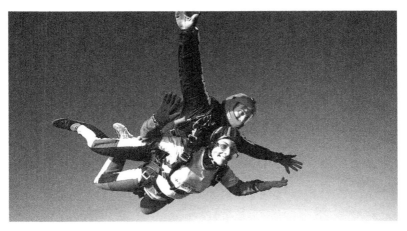

*Charity skydive, to raise funds for North West Air Ambulance,
5 months after surgery.*

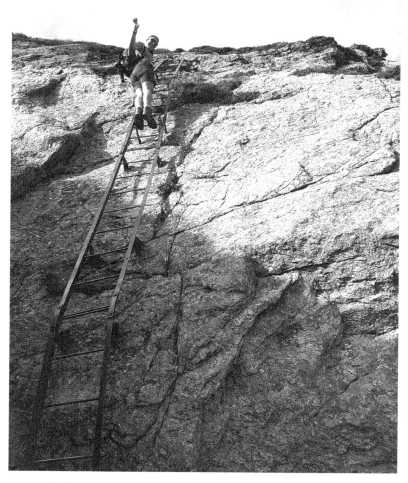

The ladder section encountered during a hike in the Alps,
5 months after surgery.

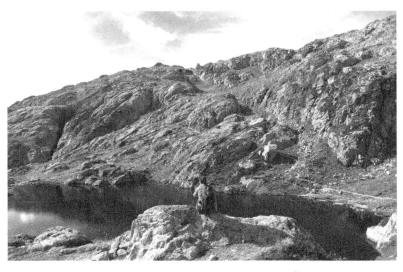

Lac Blanc, during my first trip to the Alps after surgery, October 2018.

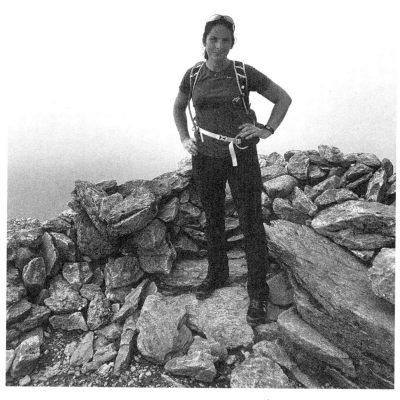

Y Garn summit, 947m, 10 weeks after surgery.

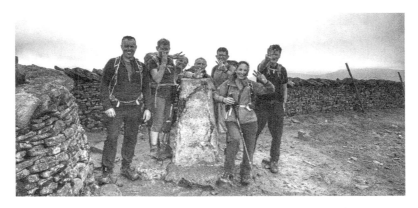

*Whernside summit, 736m, third peak on our Yorkshire
3 Peaks Challenge, a year after surgery.*

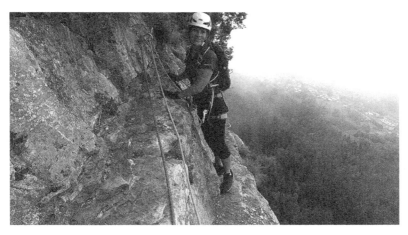

Via Ferrata in the Alps, October 2019.

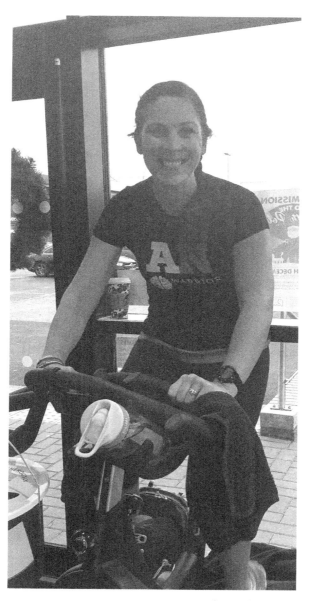

Cycling to the North Pole to raise funds for HIP (Head Injured People) in Cheshire, December 2019.

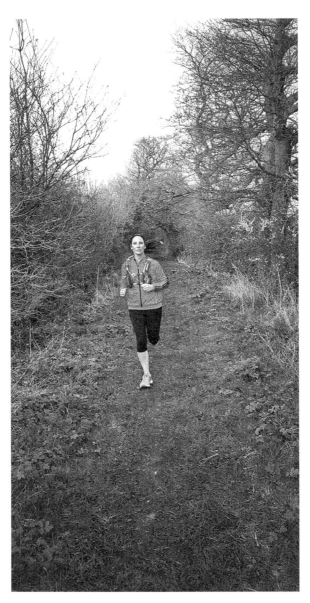

Trail running in Cheshire.

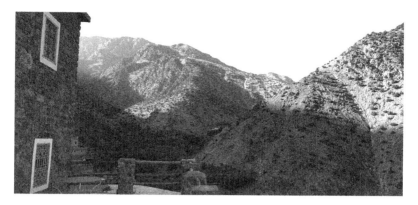

First night's accommodation in Matat village, Morocco.

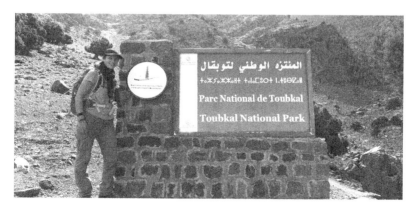

Entering Toubkal National Park.

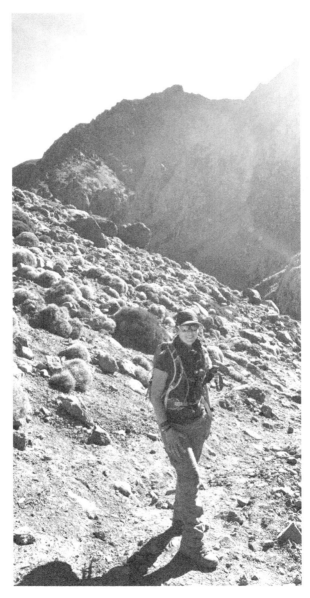

Trekking through the Atlas Mountains towards Base Camp.

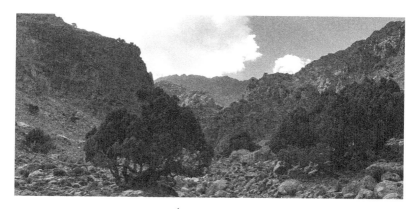

Beautiful mountain views.

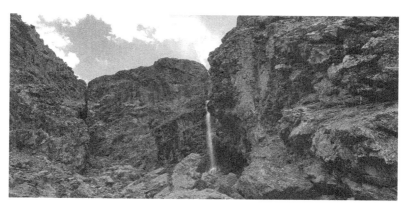

Lunch spot, sheltered away from the sun's rays.

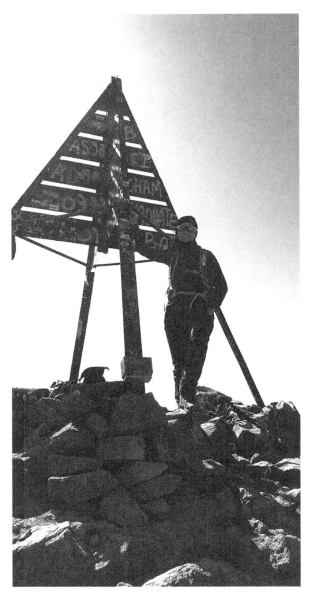

Toubkal Summit, 4167m, 1ˢᵗ October 2019.

guidance on what to expect. My first hurdle was distance, as the appointment was around 12 miles away from where I lived. It doesn't seem a big problem, but when you can't drive and you can't cope with public transport, you are reduced to begging for lifts from friends and family. Neil's place of work had been amazing and very understanding, but we were both aware that if something drastic happened, I would need him, so we tried to minimise his time off for general appointments, wherever possible. My father-in-law stepped into the breach and took me to the health centre where the assessment would take place. We sat in yet another waiting room for a few minutes before I was called in. I was rocking the pirate look, due to my eye's inability to close properly and the double vision, along with my equally dodgy shaved haircut (return to the 80s, anyone?) and clutching a wad of tissues, as I was worried about drooling from the numb corner of my mouth; I felt horribly self-conscious about discussing all of the difficulties that I experienced each day but knew it had to be done. I was reminded of my hearing loss, when I almost missed being called through, due to the assessor standing in a doorway, slightly behind me, on my deaf side, which left me feeling flustered and embarrassed. Not a great start.

I made my way into the small office, wobbling and ricocheting off the door frame, and sat myself down. I will say straight away that the assessor was a friendly man, and he did his best to put me at ease. He seemed genuinely interested in my surgery. He introduced himself as a physiotherapist and told me he'd never heard of an acoustic neuroma. He had no knowledge of my condition or the effects of surgery; that threw me – I understand that no one can know everything about every condition, but I assumed that there would be some background knowledge or research prior to the assessment. With my confused thought processes, I did my best to explain about the haemorrhage, the surgery, and the dizziness and nausea that I was still on medication for, which didn't always work. I explained that I needed support around the house, for the most basic of things; preparing meals could be an absolute minefield, as wobbling around the kitchen with sharp knives, hot surfaces and hot food, isn't ideal. I explained that I couldn't look after our children properly, and although they were doing their best to help, it was at the expense of their exams and schoolwork, which just wasn't right. I explained that I couldn't drive, and how prior to surgery I'd even got myself lost driving just 5 minutes to visit a friend – a regular journey that I had previously known as well as my own address. I informed him that I'd been instructed not to work for a minimum of 12–16 weeks from the date of my surgery, due to the serious risks of CSF leak, meningitis and so on. He diligently made notes and told me I should hear whether or not my claim was successful within a matter of weeks. As I wobbled my way back through the door, I felt a huge amount of relief that it was over, and I would likely get some financial support, which was badly needed, as my bills were mounting up and there was also the associated worry that I could do without.

It was around three weeks after the surgery that Neil went out cycling with friends for some much-needed 'me' time. When he arrived home afterwards he left his bike resting against the fence in the back garden and, after a good day, I looked at it with renewed interest. "Hmmm…" I wondered to myself. "How hard could it actually be?"

"Impossible!" Doubt declared. Not impossible, but it was hard, very hard indeed. The first difficulty was getting onto the bike; I just couldn't work out how to do it. The bike moved and I kept losing my balance. I was scared that I'd fall, end up with my head lower than it should be, and at risk of a much-feared leak. Maybe I should leave it a while? And maybe not. I thought back to how children learn, because that's exactly how I felt – like a child learning new things for the first time, but now with the added fear of failure. Neil was reluctant and quite possibly exasperated with me, but as the supportive husband he always was, he listened to my pleas and lowered the saddle. I sat on the bike. It felt so strange, and once again, almost alien to me. I cast my mind back to the first tentative walking steps I'd taken; it felt just the same and look at what had happened there...

Slowly and carefully, with my feet on the floor, I began to push myself forward along the patio. It felt as though there was a lag on my brain; it couldn't process what was happening as quickly as it needed to. After about half an hour of pushing, I thought I'd got a feel for it again, so I put one foot on a pedal, leaving the other on the floor as my safety net. The concentration it took to keep upright was incredible. It was another reminder of how much we take for granted, every single day. Again, I spent time getting used to the feeling of being back on the bike and eventually managed to get both feet off the ground. It was another victory. I really wanted to get out and try to go further, but at that moment, I was exhausted and common sense intervened. For once, I listened, knowing that this particular challenge could and would wait for another day. My mind went back into risk-assessment mode, considering the possible difficulties I could encounter. No hearing on one side was a big one; I wouldn't be able to hear where traffic was coming from and that was a major danger. I was nowhere near ready to cycle on roads yet, but I could already feel the building anxiety around this prospect. Hmmm... this was going to take some planning and measured steps, as cycling was relatively dangerous already without the added complications. Doubt didn't actually say "I told you so", but you could see that he was thinking it.

There were other problems too, I was still missing out on so many things. I missed my friends and social occasions. I missed the fun and the giggles that you can only have with good friends. Lots of meet-ups took place in the evenings because people work, and although I was still invited, I knew I'd be too exhausted to go, even though I'd done very little in the day. I didn't know how I would cope in a social setting, or indeed if I would cope. Even with my family, I struggled if there were too many voices at once, or if the television was on at the same time as someone saying something. I didn't want it to be all about me. I was worried sick that my constant refusals would mean that the invitations would stop, and I'd be forgotten. I'd already lost people that I thought the world of, and I didn't want to lose any more. There was a huge sense of urgency to get back to who I used to be.

I had suffered from anxiety in the past, or so I thought. This new, improved post-surgery anxiety was something else. I would find myself catastrophizing over everyday situations. Things that I would normally take in my stride became massive and frightening. To go from having excellent hearing, to being profoundly deaf on one side was deeply upsetting; even thinking about it made me quite angry, as it was a loss through no fault of my own. People assume that losing the hearing in one ear is just that, and you've always got the other one, but it's so much more than that. My coping mechanism was a very common one; you know that ostrich with its head in the sand? Yeah, I was right there alongside it. No matter how effective this method was, there were many times when it was just impossible to ignore. I had really enjoyed the short walks that Neil and I had achieved, increasing the distance each time and feeling very pleased with myself, but those walks were down a quiet track, in a natural environment, with very few people around. There was a little spurt of fear when Neil suggested that we ventured into town; not just town, but town on a bus.

Having spent years specialising in working with children with special needs, I really thought I knew what sensory overload was; how wrong I was. The bus itself appeared to be huge and brightly coloured. Something as simple as just walking down the aisle, between the rows of bright orange and blue seats, made me feel dizzy and nauseous. The noise of the engine seemed to be incredibly loud, and I felt as though I was sitting in the middle of it, as I couldn't work out the direction that the noise was coming from; I could feel the vibrations in my chest. The bus had announcements over a PA system, which were unbearable and grated on every nerve, despite the fact I'd placed an earplug in my good ear to take the edge off it. The lighting on the bus was harsh and searing. Despite it being a dull day, I sat there wearing my sunglasses. I couldn't wait to get off. The only thing I can liken it to is a fairground ride, one where you're hurtled forward, with disorientating lights and sounds coming from all directions. How could something as simple as a bus journey become so frightening? It would be months before I would take that trip again.

The following morning brought disappointing news. I received a letter in the post with the outcome of my PIP claim. Despite the medical evidence and advice, despite the events of the last few months since my application, and despite the obvious effects of surgery and the likelihood that I would continue to suffer for some time, if not indefinitely, a decision had been made that I wasn't ill enough, or immobile enough, to qualify for even the lower level of Personal Independence Payment, and therefore viewed as fit to work. I was so angry, frustrated and, quite frankly, hurt; it had taken a huge amount of courage to pull my senses together and to sit with a complete stranger, however nice, blurting out all of my new limitations that I was struggling to accept and trying so hard to hide in everyday life. Just how unwell did I need to be? Was a brain haemorrhage not enough? Was brain surgery that leaves you with permanent disability not enough? I felt utterly humiliated. But wait, I could appeal. Appeal? Let's not forget that I ended up in hospital with the stress of completing the initial application. Where would I get the energy and fight in order to appeal? I didn't want my life on hold for another 12 months whilst I endured an appeal process, with no guarantee of success; under the microscope and questioned, with the constant feeling of not being believed. It is a process that strips you of any shred of dignity that you might have left. I thought back to the number of cases that I'd read about, where people had found themselves in the situation I now found myself in. How I naively thought that being profoundly deaf on one side, on anti-sickness medication and with a permanently open eye, facial palsy, numbness, double vision, and balance issues, as well as being unable to drive, unable to use public transport independently, unable to cook in safety, unable to think clearly, unable to find my way around and struggling with horrendous fatigue might have been good enough reasons to claim from a system that I had paid into for most of my life, just so that in the event I'd actually need it, it would be there. It was not a lifestyle choice; it was essential. I'd even said to the assessor that I didn't want to claim a day longer than I needed to. I just wanted a little help to get through the next 12 months whilst I recovered, as best I could.

Of course, that's exactly what I should have done; I should have appealed; screamed, yelled and shown them every single issue, in glorious technicolour, but I genuinely did not have the energy, and a little bit of despair was tapping on my shoulder. Looking back at the whole thing, I think you have to consider a PIP claim as a battle; to realise that it is a long-winded process, with more steps than expected, and the appeal process is the norm for many. Instead, I took the only option I felt I had left to me, I forced myself to try and work; it was about as far from good as you can possibly get. I put myself under immense pressure for so many reasons: there was trying to get the work in, the relentless grind of advertising, the promotions, the discounts and special offers. There was the travelling to my studio; trying to arrange appointments to satisfy my clients, but also so they fitted in with when I could get lifts that didn't inconvenience people too much, and/or staying there alone for hours until Neil finished work and could pick me up. There was the putting on a front with clients, to appear as normal and professional as possible, while my brain felt as though it was wading through treacle and all I wanted to do was sleep. There was the quality of the shots; it was so difficult to assess what was good, as I really couldn't see properly, and more than once there was a 'click-and-hope-for-the-best' approach. There was the editing of the photos; there is a huge difference between editing for fun and enjoyment, and a professional edit for a client, which really does have to be breathtaking. I'm amazed that I didn't kill my fledgling business stone dead.

What you have to remember is that at that time my life was a box of complete unknowns; my specialists were saying 'We think' and 'We hope', but there were no guarantees and we were looking at a long timescale for recovery. I couldn't even make a cup of coffee, because of the boiling water and the fear I would wobble and pour it over myself. If someone made me a cup of coffee, they had to carry it for me, in case I wobbled and tipped it on myself. We really were at that level. My life was 45% worry, 45% terror and 10% incredible courage or recklessness, depending on your viewpoint. Should I have tried to ride a bike three weeks after surgery? Probably not, but I'm glad I did. Should I have gone back to work when I did? Definitely not, and I wish I hadn't, as I feel that it was detrimental to my recovery. To me, the system is badly flawed, as you have to play your best game at a time when you're potentially physically, mentally and emotionally broken. What happens to the people who have no support around them and no money? What happens to the people who are unable to fight for themselves and can see no way forward? It doesn't bear thinking about.

And oh yes… remember how the day before my surgery I'd found out that I had enlarged lymph nodes in my lungs? There could be a variety of reasons for them, but the word that stuck in my head was lymphoma. Five weeks after my surgery, I had an appointment with the respiratory consultant. He had called me at home the previous week. I couldn't help but wonder from his tone if he was speculating whether I was still around. I was booked in at the end of June, for an urgent EBUS (endobronchial ultrasound) bronchoscopy. As if I hadn't had enough hospital appointments. I was seemingly entering season ticket territory. I arrived at the hospital just after lunch. Blood was taken, blood pressure measured and recorded, cannulas inserted, and then I was sent back to the waiting room to wait my turn. My name was eventually called and I was taken through to a small theatre full of people. I lay down on the bed and they began the procedure. Once again, I've thought long and hard about whether to include this, but it is part of my story. I will warn you, it is grim, and if you need to have this done, or you're a bit squeamish, you may want to skip the next few paragraphs. I will add that the majority of people do not have this experience; I suppose I was unlucky.

As I lay back, my consultant explained that they would give me a local anaesthetic and sedative, reassuring me that most people were unable to recall the procedure after the event. I was very pleased to hear that, as it didn't sound remotely appealing. The first dose of local anaesthetic spray was administered to the back of my throat. I felt as though I was choking, but the consultant assured me that this was perfectly normal; I would still be able to swallow, and I could, but I was just unable to feel it. Really?

I was then fitted with a contraption that held my mouth open. I couldn't speak or communicate. The consultant injected more local anaesthesia into my throat, through the front of my neck, and yes, it was every bit as gross as it sounds. I was beginning to think they had forgotten about the sedative but that was the next step. As the nurse injected it through the cannula, I couldn't help thinking that it would have been better as the first step, as what had happened so far was pretty horrific. I could hear the beeping of my heart rate rapidly increasing on the monitor. My consultant and another doctor began to insert the equipment into my mouth. They explained that I might feel the urge to cough, but this was perfectly normal and I should just relax as best I could. Might? Relax? Were they kidding? Isn't that what the sedative is for?

I lay there, staring at the ceiling. I started to feel as though I was going to choke to death. I tried every distraction technique I could think of, and believe me, I knew a few; I tried counting the ceiling tiles, focusing on my feet, my two-times tables – anything that wasn't involved in this awful procedure. I felt an overwhelming urge to cough, but it wasn't the same as a normal cough, it was as though I needed to cough from my boots. I was terrified that the effort of trying to suppress it would cause my head wound to leak and I wouldn't even be able to let them know.

I couldn't understand why the sedative hadn't kicked in. I listened to the monitors beeping away and heard my blood pressure and heart rate increasing quite significantly. By this point I was coughing and choking so hard that it took three nurses to hold me down; there was one on each arm and one holding my legs. The second doctor was holding my head. I tried not to cough, but there was nothing I could do. It was on a par with being in the final stages of labour, where you have this incredible urge to push, and there's no way you can control it or stop it. My consultant asked the nurse on my left to give me another shot of sedative.

There was a moment of pure relief when he said this, and I hoped that it would mean lights out for me. Not so. I felt more alert than ever. Despite my best efforts to stay calm, this whole procedure was terrifying me and adrenaline was galloping through my veins. There was nothing I could say or do, as I was held down, with my mouth wedged open. All of them were aware of the distress I was in, and yet they continued. I began to feel as though I, as a person, didn't matter. I could feel the bronchoscopy tools poking around deep in my lungs, a sensation I never want to feel again. I was drowning. My consultant reassured me that he was almost done, there was just one more sample he needed to take, but he was struggling to get it. Finally, he got the sample and hurriedly removed the tools he'd been using. I felt horribly sick. They helped me sit upright before he told me how well I'd done and that it had gone really well. I couldn't say the same for me. I was taken back to the ward where I coughed up considerable amounts of blood. My throat felt raw, and I just wanted to get out of there as soon as I could. I felt utterly traumatised. I had been assured that it would be a simple, straightforward procedure, and that is what I prepared myself for. Nothing could have been further from the truth.

As I'd had a double dose of sedative, I was required to stay in for observation a little longer. Once the nursing team was happy, they called Neil and he came to collect me, full of comfort and reassurances. I almost ran out of the hospital, dragging him behind me; the sense of relief to be away from there was immense. There would be another week of waiting for the results.

That weekend, by way of a distraction, we decided to go for a bike ride. As usual, I did my risk assessment and chose a route that felt manageable and we were both familiar with. I was still nervous about this adventure, but we loaded the bikes into the back of the car and headed off to a point where we could pick up the cycle path. There is a café on the route that we used to visit regularly on our rides and the thought of going there again, and perhaps having a treat, was a cheering one; toasted teacake anyone? It was exhausting but so good to get back out there. I could feel my spirits soar.

One section of the route involved riding through a fairly narrow section that was fenced off on one side and had a high brick wall on the other. Just as I began to turn into this section, another couple of cyclists were heading towards us. I held my breath and hung on, feeling that I was doing ok, until the involuntary and completely uncontrollable wobbles hit. I tried desperately to stay upright, but I hadn't quite mastered that yet; I dumped myself into the fencing, giving my wrist a good crack in the process. Oh, the humiliation. Then I cried, not from the pain in my wrist, although it did hurt, but huge, gulping sobs from the hurt of losing so much. The hurt of no longer being able to enjoy a simple bike ride. The hurt of everything being so damned difficult to do and unfair. Looking back, I think there was a bit of the hurt from the hospital appointment too, and worry. I dismounted and pushed my bike along to the end of the passageway, fighting back the tears, that because of the facial palsy, still fell only from my right eye.

I was so sad that my small victory had been ripped away. Neil suggested that we went back to the car, reassuring me that it wasn't a problem if that's what I wanted to do; part of me wanted to, but that small, stubborn awkward bit (OK, not that small, but really stubborn and really, really awkward) said no. I would get to the café if it killed me, and at that point I felt there was a strong possibility that it could! As I got back onto the saddle I was shaking. My hands and wrists hurt, not only from the fall but also because I was gripping the bars so tightly. We got back onto the next section of the cycle path to continue our journey. Every turn of the pedals still felt so awkward and cumbersome; it took everything I had, and I frequently had to remind myself to breathe. Once we arrived at the coastline, the breeze picked up, adding to the challenge of staying upright. Doubt sat on the handlebars and laughed.

Eventually, we arrived at Net's Café, where thankfully there was a free table. By now, I was totally spent, to the point of speculating how I would cycle back to the car. As I sat down, I felt overwhelmed; I'd done it. I'd actually gone and done it! Yes, I felt a little wounded and my wrist was giving me moderate hell, but I had achieved what I had set out to do that morning. The feeling of accomplishment was immeasurable. I had been told to expect this to be very difficult, if not impossible. They weren't kidding. It had proved to be just as incredibly difficult as I anticipated, if not more so. There were many moments when I could have quit that ride, but I was so pleased that I'd made the decision to stick with it and carry on regardless. I'll let you into a secret. Whether through inability, or fear, many of the people who had been through the same surgery as me hadn't been able to cycle again; this knowledge had automatically moved my desire to ride a few notches up the scale, and if there was any chance at all, I was going to do it. The sense of achievement was an incredible high. Although I was aching and utterly exhausted, I couldn't wait to get back out there and ride even further. Plus, something was missing; Doubt. Oh well, he'd have to make his own way home.

The following day was results day. Neil and I arrived in a waiting room of elderly patients, the majority of whom were coughing and spluttering. Some were in wheelchairs and on oxygen, others just sat there looking frail and an unhealthy shade of grey. Not for the first time, I felt as though I didn't belong here. The wall opposite was painted red, which isn't really a calming colour for a waiting room. I gazed at the lung diagram, hung on the red wall, wondering yet again what the future would hold.

Soon enough, we were called through into a small office with a tiny window. We sat down on the uncomfortable low-backed chairs, which were becoming all too familiar, whilst the consultant presented us with the CT images of my lungs and lower abdomen. Skilfully, he pointed out the enlarged lymph nodes from which he'd taken the biopsies.

"You will be pleased to know that the results conclude that you have sarcoidosis." Sarcoidosis is an inflammatory disease, which causes patches of red and swollen tissue to form in the organs, but usually in the lungs or on the skin. It is another one that is rare. I was doing well at getting the rare stuff. I would normally have been terrified by such a diagnosis, but given what I'd already been through with the brain tumour, along with the possibility of lymphoma, this came as utter relief.

"You did really well during the procedure," he added sympathetically, to which I managed to have my say; I told him in no uncertain terms that should I ever need that barbaric procedure again, it would be under general anaesthetic. There was a pause. Finally, he advised that as the sarcoidosis was at this point showing no symptoms, he was happy to leave things as they were and monitor me. The normal treatment option would have been steroids, but I knew, and he confirmed, that the risks and side effects from their use would more than likely far outweigh any benefits. I left the hospital counting my blessings, and we headed to Manchester for the next appointment of the day.

It was my six-week post-op check-up. It was a beautiful afternoon and we arrived early for the appointment, so we bought some coffee and cake, and found a seat in the hospital grounds. We remembered how our first visit to this particular hospital had involved driving through strong winds and heavy snow, as the so-called Beast from the East hit our shores. We had been through so much since then. It was good to see Scott and Simon again. I hadn't seen Professor Lloyd since the morning after that horrific first night on the high-dependency unit, and they both commented on how good it was to see me smile. I too was relieved that I was once again able to smile, albeit ever so slightly unevenly. I'd take that, it was a lot better than it could have been. So often, we go through life taking everything for granted; having almost lost my ability to smile and losing my hearing had really underlined that. I now made a point of smiling at everyone, just because I could.

The appointment went extremely well. They inquired as to how my balance was now and I took great pleasure in telling them that I'd cycled 10 miles the previous day. I think it's fair to say that they were both impressed. I asked when I could start running again and was told they considered me to be medically fit to resume normal activities, but I should wait a little longer before getting back to climbing. Inquisitively, I asked if it would be ok for me to take part in activities at high altitudes. They confirmed that yes, I'd be fine. It was safe for me to fly and hike at high levels too. Yes! Result!

They asked about any other issues I'd had. My double vision was the same, headaches were there, but bearable and reducing in frequency; I'd even been able to come off the anti-sickness medication I'd been taking. The only issue I still had was with some of those irksome internal stitches that hadn't quite dissolved and were still pushing their way out through my wound site. They were still uncomfortable and annoying. Simon gently had a look at my wound; I was surprisingly squeamish about anyone touching it. He advised me to keep the area clean and to keep an eye on it to ensure that there were no signs of infection. He confirmed that hopefully, given time, the stitches should make their own way out; I thought it best not to tell him about the pieces of thread that I'd given a little bit of a helping hand to. Finally, I was reassured that biopsies taken from the tumour showed that it was grade 1, which was non-malignant. I would be followed up at 2, 5 and 10 years to check that there was nothing else untoward going on, as a standard procedure. For now, I could carry on working on my recovery and enjoying life.

I was, and always will be, so incredibly grateful to Scott and Simon. It is no exaggeration to say that they had given me my life back. I don't think any of us give any thought about what it could or should feel like, to come so close to death, but looking back, I think I was pretty close to finding out. Scott, Simon and the rest of the Skull Base team certainly brought me back from the brink, and from the day of my surgery, I promised myself that I would do all I could do to be grateful and live life to the full. I was going to keep that promise.

We left the hospital, both feeling elated. I wanted to celebrate by getting out for a run (I know, so rock 'n' roll), but by the time we arrived home, it was too late. To be honest, the journey and two different appointments, together with the associated stress, had taken it out of me. Running would have to wait until tomorrow.

The following day was an absolute scorcher. As soon as Neil was home from work, he drove us to the quiet lane where I had been riding my bike; it was 31 degrees and the sun beat down from a cloudless, blue sky. We set off, and once again; it just felt wrong. As the hot, late afternoon sun blazed down, I started to realise how much my head was shaken around by the running action, but it did feel good to be back out there, pounding the tarmac; maybe pounding is a little too strong, as I was trying to stay light on my feet, so my head didn't wobble too much. I was a tad apprehensive, due the ever-present fear of a CSF leak. As I looked forward, objects were moving around far more than I ever remembered; I felt as though my eyes were jumping around in my head.

We clocked up 3.5 kilometres in around half an hour. Although I realised how much fitness I'd lost in six months, I was still absolutely delighted. Doubt popped up and asked if I really thought I'd ever be as fit as I used to be; I ignored him. I was just so happy to be there (in more ways than one) and happy to be running at all. Holding hands, Neil and I strolled back to the car where we stopped, chatted and cooled off a little before driving home. Despite the high, I was exhausted once again.

The following weeks comprised of walking as much as I could, fitting in a couple more runs, and spending a considerable amount of time lounging around, crashing out on the sofa or in the garden. It was a boom–bust cycle. Admittedly, there were times it felt significantly more bust than boom. During those first few weeks, I could endure the process by considering it to be my body doing what it needed to do in order to fully recover. As the weeks and months went by, mentally, it became much harder to justify the sleep time, and it was starting to feel like a backward step. This wasn't helped by having to go back to work. I had taken a couple of bookings that I was determined to honour. I couldn't afford not to, as the bills were still rolling in. The first was a cake smash. How difficult could it really be? It was a minefield. First of all, I had to enlist Neil's help to set up the backdrops, as I still shouldn't lift anything heavy. Then there was the matter of blowing up balloons. I couldn't do this either, due to the pressure it would put on my head. Again, Neil got the job. As for the session itself, well I must have looked like I had a rod down my back as I sat on the floor, terrified of bending down, just in case… I had been in a dilemma as to whether or not I should tell my clients what was going on. I felt that once it was out, I couldn't take it back, and perhaps they would just find someone else to do their photoshoot. I valued every one of my clients, and was determined not to let this happen, so I just kept quiet. Whilst the session went well, I really struggled with the editing side of the business. Looking at the computer seemed to just suck the life force out of me, and I would be unable to edit for more than half an hour at a time.

Sunday, 8th July. Eight weeks and one day after my surgery. It was another scorching summer's day, with a glorious deep blue sky; the early morning sun shone down on us. We made our way to Chester Racecourse, with my friend Sahra, who had decided to run with me; I don't think Sahra had run since high school, and I'm pretty certain that she was starting to regret the offer, which made me appreciate it and her even more. It was my first post-surgery race, and I felt sick with a mix of nervous anticipation and excitement. There was such a great atmosphere, and this year, for obvious reasons, the event was particularly poignant for me. Music blasted out from the stage area, whilst people of all ages milled around in a sea of smiles and pink. It really was my race for life. This event had been my original goal, back in the early days of my diagnosis. I couldn't believe that the day had finally arrived, and I was able to run at least some, if not all of it!

As the race started, I found it quite challenging (understatement) to stay in a straight line, with so many people around me. Sahra stuck by my side, and each time I drifted off course, I felt a hefty tug, as she pulled me back on track; not only was the poor woman running when she wasn't used to it, but she must have felt as though she was trying to herd a particularly ambitious toddler. It was so incredibly hot that morning; on a couple of occasions I felt dizzy and nauseous, which brought fears of was it my head or was I just a bit dehydrated? I wasn't sure. I stayed in what little shade there was and kept drinking. We slowed down to a walk, with Sahra by my side, until the feeling subsided; I am so grateful to that woman, for everything. Crossing that finish line and claiming my finisher's medal was amazing! I had such a feeling of accomplishment. I had survived something that sadly some others hadn't. I'd reclaimed a significant part of my life, where some others hadn't. I was hungry for more.

As we stood for photos, my mind began to whirl, but in a good way. This had been my target, my goal. At times I had questioned whether I would get here at all, but I had, and not only that, I'd completed it. So, what now? The Race for Life had been my focus for months. What was the motivation now? I was going to have to give it some serious thought. I wanted to stay and savour the moment, but Neil was keen to get out of the heat and beat the traffic, so we headed for home. Looking back, I think he was concerned that I'd pushed myself too hard, as he understood the fatigue side of things. If only he knew the thoughts going through my head for what I could do next.

It wasn't long before my next challenge fell into my lap; Chester Great Outdoors Club, which we had joined just months before this nightmare began, were planning a hike in Snowdonia. There would be just a couple of weeks to wait. Whilst Mount Snowdon is the highest peak in this national park, forming a prominent position in the centre of the Snowdon Horseshoe, the peak and its surrounding slopes are prime examples of extreme glaciation, bearing all the tell-tale signs of the wild landscape's vibrant past. Alluvial fans line the steep slopes of the glacial lakes, with the only evidence of a long-gone Ice Age being the rocky debris littering the land. It could be a busy place, full of families visiting for the day, walkers, climbers and hikers, but I still loved its vast wilderness. It's a credit to Neil that when I told him what I was planning to do this time, he didn't really flinch; well, maybe he did, just a bit.

The outing was to be a short, scrambling route on mixed terrain. It was an area I had previously visited, and I immediately wanted to do it, but as the day got closer, doubts began to creep in. I found myself obsessing over videos of the route, scrutinizing the ground and the rocks, and wondering if I could actually do it. Doubt pointed out that it would be the most challenging route I'd taken on for quite some time, and he thought it was out of my reach. I had to flip my thinking, and quick, before I listened to Doubt. I still watched the videos, but rather than looking for hazards that I might struggle with, I visualised myself on the route; I imagined what each step would feel like, and how, despite the ground being uneven, I would take each step confidently. Most importantly of all, I would stay upright.

When the day arrived, I felt queasy with nerves, but once I started chatting to the others, that feeling subsided and we began our walk. The first section took us across a grassy track around a lake called Llyn Idwal. The scenery was so beautiful, and I stopped for a moment just to take it in and appreciate it; this is what I'd missed. As we followed the edge of the lake, we were surrounded by impressive, rocky peaks. The bright sunlight glinted on the still surface of the lake, whilst magnificent birds of prey circled overhead, using the warm air to rise even higher. I took a deep breath and moved on.

The undulating, grassy ground gave way to small rocks and till, and we soon picked our way onto a path up towards the Devil's Kitchen. Slipping and sliding, I found it noticeably tougher than it had ever been before, and I soon tired with the constant need to correct my balance to stay upright, as it was no longer instinctive. I used the bigger boulders for support, scanning for suitable handholds; the relentless movement of my head looking up and down made me feel queasy, but I kept going.

Kept pushing on. Doubt reminded me that I didn't have to do this and a rest would be nice. I ignored him.

People often use the analogy of how swans glide gracefully across water, whilst beneath the surface, their feet are frantically paddling away; that was exactly how I felt. My body was screaming for me to stop, but I just wanted to hide the battle that was going on; to appear normal to everyone else. It was a case of stop, start, stop, start, all the while pretending to myself, and others, that I wasn't struggling. That I wasn't feeling as though I was going to throw up at any moment. That I wasn't having to make any more effort than most. It was hot, I was incredibly tired, and I just wanted to lie down and sleep.

As we emerged from Devil's Kitchen, we found ourselves shrouded in cloud, so we made our way to the edge of a small glacial lake. In the mist, it was noticeably cooler, so all the layers I'd taken off during my ascent soon went back on. I took a deep lungful of the clean, cool air, and admired the beauty of the rock formations that surrounded us, calming myself, and regaining my equilibrium. It felt so good to be back out with like-minded people, doing what I loved.

I sat there, thinking how just 10 weeks earlier, my long surgery had just started; my surgeons must have been concerned, as they'd later admitted they had no idea what they'd find, because of the potential damage that the haemorrhage may have caused. "Get me back to the mountains…" Well, they'd certainly done that. I thought of how impossibly difficult those early hours and days were, how I thought I'd never be able to get to places like this again. It's hard not to get caught up in those feelings of despair. It was frightening to think back to these life-changing events, knowing that my outcome could have been so very, very different. Even at wonderful, long-awaited moments such as this, the negative thoughts intruded.

We packed up and started our ascent of the mountain Y Garn. The air became warm, thick and humid; the path we were following was gravelly and fairly good underfoot, but steep. I pressed on, but soon tiredness was nibbling at my heels. I began to fall back. Pacing myself is something that has never come naturally; I've always been an all-or-nothing kind of person, yet here I was being forced to slow down; to approach things in a different way. I can't say I was a fan of that, in any way, shape or form.

The summit of Y Garn is fairly unremarkable, compared to others, but reaching that landmark for me was a milestone in so many ways. The last six months had been a huge journey; at times it was painful, upsetting and soul-destroying, but it had also contained huge amounts of self-discovery. I had been to places I never knew existed for me. Places so heartbreakingly dark that I never wanted to visit them again. I had experienced highs and lows, but the lows tallied the greatest number. I had felt so challenged and empty; there were times I really didn't know if I would make it. Nevertheless, here I was standing on top of a mountain, a 947-metre mountain, to be precise. Yes, there was thick cloud and no views to speak of, but at that moment in time, I was on top of the world. I stood there and savoured the moment with my friends and then hung back to enjoy the moment alone.

In the lead up to this, Doubt had practically been my constant companion, his little voice telling me what I could, and more frequently what I couldn't, do. The thing is that visualisation is a powerful and often underused tool. Some of the time, I could ignore the negative noise and instead focus on seeing myself doing the things I wanted to do. Admittedly, my visualisation skills needed some work, but it was a step in the right direction. Funnily enough, I never had a problem with visualising giving Doubt a kick up the butt.

The warm, humid air was almost totally still and I was brought back to the present moment by a swarm of black flies that had decided to settle on my bare arms and another group of hikers about to reach the summit.

Still feeling a sense of elation, and not wanting to leave that glorious moment in time, I gathered my thoughts and my gear together and began the seemingly never-ending, rocky descent back towards Llyn Idwal. Thankfully, despite tired legs, there were none of the slips, trips or falls that I had been dreading, and with that, and a newfound sense of achievement, we loaded the car up and headed back over the border to England.

CHAPTER 5

We were blessed with yet another warm, sunny morning. I was enjoying a coffee, which was now tasting more like it should do, and scrolling through a social media page when it appeared on my newsfeed…

Would you be willing to take to the skies for North West Air Ambulance? Book a skydive now for just £50.

I thought back to my meeting with Scott and Simon; they'd said I would be fine to do activities at altitude, but were they thinking skydive when they said that? I clicked *Book Now*.

In those few months after my surgery, my life was a strange combination of highs and lows, with usually more lows, although there was a consistent thread of gratitude running through it all. To go from being almost totally bed-bound and quite literally expecting a quick knock on the door from the Grim Reaper, to getting your life back to a point where it wasn't a million miles from normal, had given me a new sense of purpose. I wanted to be able to give something back. I briefly read through the terms and conditions, the usual health declaration stuff, and thought maybe I could get away with the disclaimer, as there was nothing *specific* to my experience. With no time like the present, I set up my funding page there and then, and waited.

Neil and I had a much-needed holiday booked, and we set off for a glorious week on the beautiful Greek island of Kos. As the sun bounced into our apartment, my phone began to ring on the dressing table. I answered to find it was the lady from the charity's fundraising team... she had read my story on my fundraising page and wanted to check that I'd been medically cleared to take part.

"Of course," I replied, with conviction. Damn, had my plans been scuppered already? As soon as I was off the phone, I searched through my emails to find the one she'd already sent through with the medical forms attached, and forwarded them to Scott Rutherford's secretary, with my fingers crossed! Better late than never...

Our Greek island holiday was amazing. My senses had been heightened and I became far more aware of things I might otherwise have taken for granted: walking barefoot on sand, the heat of the sun on my skin, the blueness of the sky, and the sound of the waves breaking on the shore. Once again, I was reminded of how good it was to be alive.

The only thing to mar my happiness was my hearing loss. Single-sided or unilateral hearing loss comes with a whole host of problems that you would find hard to imagine. Yes, I still have one ear that works, but localising sound is problematic at best, not to mention the great difficulty understanding speech in noisy surroundings. Bars and restaurants were particularly challenging. I lost count of the number of times I was caught out by the waiter standing behind me or on my wrong side, waiting for me to give him my order. I felt so embarrassed and thought that I must look rude to them. There were a few workarounds we employed. We now thought very carefully about where we sat; at the hotel, I would sit, wherever possible, with my bad ear facing toward the road, and my good ear in toward the restaurant. This was great for blocking out the noisy mopeds, quad bikes and buggies, but not so great with the noise of everyone chatting away in my good ear. Neil must have been fed up with hearing me ask, "What did you say?". I was equally fed up with his response, "It doesn't matter". It did matter. It mattered to me. I wanted to be included, to be a part of the conversation.

After dinner and a few cocktails at a nearby bar, we would retreat to the quieter seafront, where in my now usual style of turning obstacles into challenges, I would entertain both Neil and myself by seeing just how much alcohol would compromise my already compromised vestibular system. In the dark, feeling tired, wearing flip-flops, and fuelled by strawberry daiquiris (all the things I had been warned would make balance difficult) I would step onto the low sea wall and see how far I could go, before wobbling off onto the sand, or I would walk along the kerbstones with my arms flailing, as though walking a tightrope. Surprisingly, the practice each night led to incremental improvements, so to challenge myself further, I would then attempt (often unsuccessfully) the yoga tree pose. I wonder if our physios will ever recognise the flip-flop and strawberry daiquiri method of therapy. I can highly recommend it.

Some of my life had certainly changed, and changed in a big way. I could see that I would just have to get used to making alterations to the way I now did things; as much I didn't want to, frustratingly, it was necessary. As someone who loved going out and socialising, hearing loss had taken away much of the enjoyment that I once knew. People just didn't seem to understand how so much of day-to-day life could be affected when I still had one ear that worked well. It was hard to explain and I'm certain they thought I was making excuses. For instance, unilateral hearing loss meant I could no longer localise a sound. If someone called me from down the street, I would have no idea which direction they were calling from. When it happened, I would often cope by just completely ignoring them. I know this must have appeared to be really rude sometimes, but I hoped that people would just put it down to my deafness; to respond would mean that I'd have to spin around, trying not to fall over in the process, while desperately looking in all directions for someone I might know.

Hearing over background noise was now almost impossible. In a noisy bar, for example, everything seemed to be the same volume – just think about that for a moment; everyone talking, the music, the clattering glasses, plates and cutlery, the chairs scraping on the tiled floor, and the person I was sat just two feet away from, all at the same volume. It was and still is very frustrating.

As a distraction in these circumstances, my thoughts turned to my skydive and I became focused on raising as much as possible for the North West Air Ambulance, an extremely worthwhile charity. No one knows when they may need an air ambulance; I was astounded to discover many years ago that they're not run by the NHS or the government, although the NHS provide the clinical staff and the equipment – they rely on charitable donations for day-to-day operations. As the big day approached, in true British style the weather began to take a turn for the worse. I watched the forecasts religiously and with a storm due in on the weekend of the jump, rather angrily I convinced myself that it wouldn't go ahead. I sat waiting by the computer for the notification ping that would put an end to my prolonged misery: it never came.

The skydive was due to take place on Sunday 14th October, but on the 12th and 13th, Storm Callum hit our shores, forecast to impact large parts of the country, particularly across the west of the UK. The skydive was to take place in Lancaster, and you can't really get more westerly than that. I woke that morning to dark, menacing skies and a feeling of extreme disappointment. It was still windy, but not quite as bad as the previous two days. I couldn't imagine the jump taking place in this weather, so I called the skydive centre to ask if it was still worth me turning up. The reply was most definitely yes, come along as planned.

They confirmed that the forecast had shown an improvement from lunchtime, so in disbelief we set off and headed north to Lancaster. As the wind buffeted the car, I still wasn't convinced that it could possibly go ahead. Doubt laughed; his opinion was 'absolutely no chance', and it would be a wasted journey.

As we left the motorway, the sky was heavy with clouds and red and gold leaves were falling like colourful rain from the trees. How on earth could this go ahead? Then I saw it – a tiny sliver of blue in the distance. It was so tiny, it could easily have been missed, but it gave me the first glimmer of hope that perhaps this jump might just happen. As Neil navigated our way through a number of small villages, I became transfixed on the tiniest glimmer of bright blue cutting sharply through the foreboding rainclouds. The closer we got to the skydive centre, the brighter the sky became, and for the first time I began to feel excited. The parachute centre was a group of buildings, set well off the beaten track, in the middle of farmland. The gloomy skies were being replaced with rays of sunshine breaking enthusiastically through the clouds. As I looked skyward, I saw a light aircraft circling above. Moments later, I could just about make out a small door being opened and people started to jump, their chutes opening about a minute later. It was amazing to see. I realised with a punch of excitement that I would soon be one of those people, floating gracefully back to earth.

The previous year during a trip to Chamonix in the French Alps, before life as I knew it was flipped upside down, Neil and I had been paragliding. It was an incredible experience; we had taken a cable car to Plan de l'Aiguille at 2,317 metres altitude, followed by a short walk to a designated area for taking off. It didn't take too long for us to be strapped firmly into our harnesses, fastened securely to our tandem instructors and told how we should quite simply run off the mountainside and keep running until we were told to stop. You really couldn't go wrong.

Weather-wise, it had been a similar sort of day too. We had woken to dark heavy cloud clinging to the valley and, again, I was expecting it to be cancelled. By late morning, however, the veil of cloud began to thin; we were blessed with bright sunshine and the most incredible views as we glided high above the mountains. From up high, I saw ibex warming themselves on rocks in the sunshine. I grabbed my camera and took as many photographs as I could from this incredible viewpoint. The trees were beginning to change their colour from green to autumnal reds and golds, and the fresh, unpolluted air was both tranquil and quiet. As we drifted over the town, I remember sounds becoming clearer; I could hear the train, children playing, workmen drilling, but overall, I just remember how peaceful it all was.

I had imagined my skydive would be a similar experience. Handing over my now signed medical form, I registered myself at the reception, before the dreaded task of weighing in. I had registered to jump from 11,000 ft, but was offered the chance to upgrade to 15,000 ft. I mean, you still have to get out of the door, right? I also booked a videographer, Leroy, to film the event; for me this was a once-in-a-lifetime experience that at one point I thought I'd never be able to do; I wanted to hang on to those precious memories.

We talked through what would happen that day and then went to wait outside in the now glorious sunshine. It was beautiful, but quite cool, and we spent some time watching others land in the field. There was a huge puddle right next to the landing zone; good job I wasn't in charge of the steering, as I was pretty sure we'd be landing in the middle of it!

There was a buzz of excitement in the air. I was so glad to see that many others were jumping for North West Air Ambulance that afternoon, and I finally met up with Linda, the fundraising lady who had called me about the medical form. When my name was called, I went through to a large room where one of the instructors, Ben, gave a presentation on procedure and health and safety. He was confident and funny, soon putting everyone at ease. It was a fast-paced run-through, as the weather had made the day's schedule very tight, and the instructors were keen to get through as many jumps as they could.

Looking back, I still don't think the realisation of what I was about to do had sunk in. Once again, we were asked to wait outside to hear who our tandem jump instructors would be; it turned out that mine would be Ben. I was glad, as he was one of those reassuring individuals who immediately put you at ease, plus, as I've previously said, he was funny. He took me back inside and fitted me out with an over suit, gloves and an oh-so-gorgeous hat! I looked like Buzz Aldrin about to board the Saturn V for a lunar landing – was it too late to cancel the videographer? He asked if I was nervous at all, and I firmly replied no; actually, I was feeling a surreal sense of calm. The only thing that bothered me was the thought of not being able to hear his instructions. There's a time to hide things and pretend that everything is normal. Yeah, this wasn't it; I told him my worry and so calmly and reassuringly, he went over everything again.

It wasn't much of a wait until we boarded the small aircraft. It was unlike any plane I'd ever been in, and was more like sitting in the back of a van with wings! Absolutely no luxury here! There were no seats, just two benches running down each side, and there was certainly no prospect of duty free. We were sitting very snuggly, our legs straddling the benches, and once everyone was in place, we began to taxi across the small airfield before taking off. The views over the coastline were amazing and, apart from a few tufts of cotton wool clouds, the sky was now a glorious blue above us. It's amazing how much the weather can change in just a few hours.

As we reached 7,000 ft, the instructors began attaching themselves to our harnesses and performing safety checks on each other. I struggled to hear over the noise of the engines and people chatting, but there was a great atmosphere with lots of fun banter and nervous laughter going on. I gazed out of the small window taking in the views, as we continued to climb. My mouth was dry, quite possibly due to the adrenaline rush that was going on, but in part due to the after-effects of surgery. Minutes later, the roller door was opened and the temperature plunged as the cold air rushed in. The cabin soon began to empty as two-by-two, people slid their way down the benches, sat on the floor and then pushed themselves out. It was strange to see people disappearing out of the door of a moving aircraft.

Being first into the plane meant we were the last out. We slid along the bench, dropped onto the floor and then sat for a moment taking in the views. It was surreal. There was absolutely nothing between me and the colourful patchwork of fields a mile below. As I'd been instructed, I tucked my legs under the aircraft, and leaned back tilting my head up. Before I knew it, we were suddenly out in the open. Those first few seconds felt strange and disorientating. As we left the plane, we seemed to be plunging almost headfirst towards the ground. I focussed entirely on keeping my legs bent, as instructed, and we soon levelled off. Ben tapped me on my shoulder as a sign that I could release my arms from my chest strap, but I had wedged my thumbs so tightly behind them that I struggled to get them out. I had expected that my stomach would turn somersaults, but strangely, and thankfully, it didn't.

We were free falling at around 120 mph and the air roared down my hearing ear. Suddenly, Leroy appeared; again, it seemed totally unimaginable that you could be 15,000 ft up in the air, with nothing between you and the ground below, and then you see a fellow human being just suspended there in front of you. He had a camera attached to his helmet, taking stills with a control operated by his teeth I think, and a GoPro camera taking video footage.

After 60 seconds of free fall, Ben released the chute. We suddenly jolted, as though someone had put the brakes on, and my legs dropped. The roaring noise stopped suddenly and I was struck by just how quiet it was.

"How was that?" asked Ben. It was quite possibly the most awesome experience I'd ever had. I think it beat my covert night-time trip on a Navy rib in the straits of Gibraltar some years ago, but that's another story and one that probably shouldn't be told!

Now it was quiet, we recapped our landing procedure. When Ben gave the instruction 'Legs up!' I would lift my legs using the handles in the legs of my oversuit, so I would be in a mid-air sitting position, then he would do the rest. We would come to land on our backsides. Sounded pretty simple, although I was still mindful of that big puddle. Slowly, we descended whilst Ben gave me a guided tour of the area, pointing out features such as the Lancaster Canal, and other landmarks like the Blackpool Tower glistening in the late-afternoon, autumnal sunshine. It was another world, a world of tranquillity and solitude. A world where my hearing wasn't an issue because there was no noise. It was a world a part of me didn't want to leave.

Roughly five minutes later, we approached the landing zone. Although I was still acutely aware that part of the field was submerged under a large puddle, due to the extensive rainfall that there had been over the previous few days, I had every faith that Ben would bring us down away from it. As the ground moved closer towards us, it gave the illusion we were speeding up, and I wondered if we would overshoot the landing strip. I could see Leroy, already down on the ground and ready to film our landing. Then came the instruction "Legs up, legs up, legs up!" so I did as I was told and we slid along the well-worn, muddy grass.

It was utterly amazing. Exhilarating! My heart was still racing as I was asked by our cameraman what I'd thought of the experience. I had genuinely loved every single moment; from the flight, to the freefall, to the ride down and the landing. I would have gone back up there in a heartbeat.

My fear and anxiety of not being able to hear had, on this occasion, been totally unfounded. I think my biggest fear was actually admitting that I struggled with it, but once I'd explained to people, they would be totally understanding and accommodating of the fact. Ben had just taken it in his stride and it was no big deal. I wish I could say the same.

At the other end of the fear spectrum, my fear threshold of physical challenges was becoming considerably higher than those around me, no doubt as a direct result of having gone through the ordeal of my surgery, along with everything leading up to it. In fact, my relationship with fear was becoming a strange one, one that friends and family found hard to understand. As I see it, I can let fear paralyse me, and stop me from enjoying life, or I can use it as my motivation. After all, what is fear? Does it actually exist, or is it something we create in our minds?

CHAPTER 6

Throwing myself out of a plane was the most incredible experience, but as the days went by and my adrenaline returned to normal levels, I found myself feeling a little deflated. It happens – like anything that you've spent ages preparing for, it leaves a huge gap when it's gone.

Following my seemingly rapid recovery from surgery, we decided to go back to the Alps, for several reasons; it was a place we loved, but it also completed the circle of me being healthy, diagnosis, treatment, recovery, and finally being healthy again. It was almost symbolic if you like. The village of Chamonix is nestled at an altitude of 1,035 m, to the north of Mont Blanc, the highest summit in the Alps. It sits between the peaks of Aiguille Rouge and Aiguille du Midi. Hiking up the sides of the valley is rewarded with incredible panoramic views. Not only was it an amazing place to hike, but the town itself had a great atmosphere; full of friendly locals and tourists, all sharing a love of this beautiful, rugged environment. I was feeling happy and optimistic, with no trace of Doubt at all. I certainly didn't want him and his luggage tagging along.

Ahead of our trip, we spent hours researching routes we hadn't hiked before, making plans, downloading maps, and checking out local transport routes and connections. I was confident that all of this would be within my grasp, and although I realised that it could be tiring, it still felt manageable. A week or so after the skydive, we departed from Manchester Airport to Geneva, Switzerland, from where we would make the hour-long journey to our hotel in Chamonix. So far, so good. Our first trip of the holiday involved a bus ride out to the hamlet of Montroc, from where we picked up our path, which would take us up to Lac Blanc. The initial section of the path led us through beautiful woodland, with stunning views of the Mont Blanc Massif across the valley. It was wonderfully exhilarating to be out there again, and I felt so incredibly thankful to be alive.

I had taken my camera and stopped frequently to admire the view and take photos of anything that caught my eye. My camera had become another coping mechanism; it was my way of taking a quick breather when fatigue was becoming a problem, without letting others know that I was struggling. It had felt distinctly cool that morning, and so we had set out wearing long trousers and down jackets. The long steep climb through the woodland had soon warmed us up, though, and it wasn't long before we found ourselves delayering and swapping the long trousers for shorts!

Frustratingly, I was having to take more frequent breaks and I was finding the climb harder than I had in the past, and certainly far harder than expected. I was struggling with the unfamiliar, uneven paths and I was feeling nauseous. Step by step, we kept moving forward, Neil reassuring me that it wouldn't be much further until we reached the top, from where we would just follow the contour before heading over to Lac Blanc.

I insisted on checking the map; as much as I love him, Neil is one of those irritating people who will say you don't have too far to go, when in fact you have miles and miles ahead of you! We were approaching a section on the map that looked incredibly steep; in fact, there seemed to be no gaps at all between the contour lines. Doubt suddenly piped up with, "You can't do that!" I kept on looking; as much I hate to say it, I had to agree with him. It looked far too steep for me.

We'd come this far already, so we decided to press on and see what this next stretch looked like. Little did we realise, this was a ladder section and there was no way around it. The only way was up. Looking back, I'm not sure whether it was a good or bad thing that we didn't realise in advance that there was such a technical section. Part of me thinks that if I'd known there was, I would have avoided this route. I was now in a situation where I'd found the incline quite tiring already and was almost glad of the ladders, as that meant we could make a quick ascent. With that, I kicked Doubt off the first rung and took my first step up. It was another first, as I'd not tried anything this technical post-surgery. Could I do it? You bet I could!

It was a relief to finally reach the highest point of the route before we followed the contour along towards the lake. As we rounded the final corner, the glistening blue waters of Lac Blanc came into view. The tiredness and the angst of the ladder climbing soon melted away, as I took in the beauty and tranquillity of my surroundings. I found myself a boulder on which to sit, overlooking the magnificent lake; the clear blue sky above and the silhouette of the mountains reflected in the smooth glass-like surface of the crystal-clear water, as the sun beat down on us. It was truly breathtaking. I could see flowers and was struck by how even in the most inhospitable of places beautiful flowers still bloomed between the sharp rocks; a metaphor for life, and a reminder that growth happens even in the harshest of environments. Despite feeling physically broken by this point, I had still progressed further than I ever thought I would, in just a few months.

Once I'd sat down, though, I didn't want to move; I could quite happily have found myself a sheltered spot to try to get some sleep. Thankfully, Neil kept me awake and as soon as we'd eaten lunch, we continued on our way. I was now having to dig deep into what little energy reserves I had remaining. The path began to drop down, and I slipped a few times on tired legs, each slip causing a jarring, jolting sensation to my balance, and that quick squirt of adrenaline from thinking that you're going to fall. I had badly underestimated just how exhausted I would feel at altitude and was overwhelmed by a mix of emotions, which are always worse when you're fatigued.

It's strange how emotions work; no matter what, I was happy that I had made it back to these beautiful mountains, but I was also angry, resentful and upset that the enjoyment from this adventure that should have been mine had been tempered by the fatigue and nausea I was now experiencing. I was certain that my life was never meant to be like this. I resented the fact that after the tumour all spontaneity had gone. Everything now involved well-thought-out plans, with exit strategies, plan Bs and sometimes plan Cs. I was constantly overthinking what lay ahead. Doubt floated along beside me singing, "I told you so".

We had planned to track along the ridge, before dropping back down into Chamonix, but my energy levels were utterly depleted, and it was time to reluctantly admit defeat, which never sits well with me. We made it to La Flégère and took the decision to take the cable car down, and then take a bus back into town.

I really had wanted to walk. I wanted to put the miles in that day, in a place I loved. I resented the fact that I was the cause of our plans having to change; even though I knew it was something that was out of my hands, it didn't help. There was a long queue waiting for the cable car, and having spoken to the attendant, I discovered it was the last one down off the mountain that day. Something must have shown in my face, as the attendant was very sympathetic, allowing us to board without tickets, asking only that we pay when we got to the ticket office at the bottom. With that, we squashed in and headed down into the valley. I looked on as the zigzag path we should have taken down through the woodland disappeared from sight. From up above, it was easy to think I'd made the wrong decision, and we should have walked, but the reality was it was much further and steeper than it looked, and there would have been a strong possibility that my ride back to town might have been an ambulance, rather than the bus!

The bus ride was a quiet one. Too tired to speak, I became lost in my bleak thoughts, as around me young children chatted with each other about their school day, and Doubt looked smug as he crossed his arms and rested his feet on the seat in front. I was far too exhausted to become emotional. Once we reached our stop, we took the short stroll back to the hotel. I threw myself onto the bed and slept.

The contingency plans we made meant that we would hire a couple of bikes the following day, to have a more relaxing and easier time exploring the forest trails. I was looking forward to a day of sitting down, using two wheels rather than my feet. We picked our mountain bikes up early the next morning, heading off in the direction of the River Arve, which runs through the valley.

We had planned to make our way to the forest trails, explore for a while and then head back into town at the end of the day, but just 10 minutes into the ride I felt so awful I just wanted to go back and hand the bike in at the shop. Instead, we pushed on. I struggled with everything for so much of that day. My head felt like it was in a washing machine, on a spin cycle. Feelings of nausea washed over me in waves, and as time went on, I felt any shreds of confidence I had left evaporate away through my clammy skin.

As we reached the trails, a local cyclist insisted on telling me my saddle was too low. He meant well of course, and I knew it was low, but I couldn't be bothered to explain the intricacies of my surgery there and then, in French, so when he finally got the message that I was happy with my saddle in the position it was, he shrugged his shoulders, huffed and puffed a little, then continued on his way. The inclines were impossible for me, as due to the reduction in speed as I went uphill I consequently lost momentum. I had neither the balance nor the energy to keep going. I cannot recall how many times I went crashing to the floor, only to get up and get back on the bike again. The down-hill sections were nothing short of terrifying, as I felt completely out of control, my brain seemingly unable to process what was going on at speed. Double vision didn't help with looking out for rocks and tree roots; on my left side I felt like I was watching a 3D film, without the glasses. Somewhere deep inside my head was a roaring sound, whilst wind noise overwhelmed my hear-ing ear. Time and time again I fell off, getting so battered and bruised that everything hurt, including my pride, which would take significantly longer to heal. I spent more time pushing my bike than cycling. The nausea I felt now was on a whole new level. Neil didn't know what to say or what to do, as he has always tried to encourage me and be supportive, but this was uncharted territory for both of us. I'm embarrassed to say that at one point I dismounted and angrily threw my bike to the ground; a proper temper tantrum, driven by frustration, worthy of a two-year-old. Even Doubt kept quiet.

We were out in the middle of nowhere, so again I forced us into taking the decision to change our planned route, choosing to stay on a low level and flat. We made our way to a small hamlet and picked up a quiet road that took us most of the way back to Chamonix, where we followed the glacial blue waters of the Arve back to town. Even that route was problematic, as riding on the right side of the road now meant that my deaf ear was on the side of any approaching traffic. My anxiety was through the roof and it felt as though a jet engine was roaring away in my head. Several times I had to just stop, take a few deep breaths and ground myself before continuing. It was hard on so many levels.

We got back to our hotel mid-afternoon, much earlier than planned, and I threw myself on the bed and slept for hours. I realise now this was due to the physical demands the cycling had taken on my vestibular system. You see, my body now has to put in twice as much mental and physical effort and energy to stay upright, if not more. I was completely and utterly exhausted, not helped by the raging anger I felt towards myself. It was very easy to forget that just 5 months earlier I could barely even walk...

Our final day of hiking in the Alps was a similar story. We took a cable car up to Plan de l'Aiguille, from where we were going to follow the ridge along to Mer du Glace, intending to take the train from there back down to the bottom of the valley. As we set off along the undulating trail from the lift station, we were chatting with a couple of guys who were visiting from the United States; actually, it was Neil who was talking to them, whilst I began to fall further and further behind. True to form, it wasn't long before I stumbled and fell, tearing my favourite trousers and cutting my knee. I was too tired for tears and tantrums, but I was angry with everyone and everything; I was especially angry with me.

We hadn't even covered half of our planned route when Neil took control (brave man). He decided we needed to turn back and head for the lift station to take the cable car back down. He told me in no uncertain terms that the speed I was going at would have meant we were likely to miss the last train down, and he wasn't prepared to do that. He was right. Of course, he was right, but I felt defeated, and at that point a complete and utter failure. Doubt had a field day rejoicing in my misfortune. From the outset, I was adamant that I would not accept a new normal unless I had absolutely no other choice, and yet here I was struggling like hell to just do normal, let alone hiking in the Alps. Looking back, that trip was the start of a very steep, unpleasant learning curve for me.

I have always been driven and goal-focussed, and more often than not I have been very successful with that approach. The trouble was that this approach was no longer working for me in the way that it once had. If I were honest, it was working against me. Before my surgery, someone had said that the way forward was to improvise, adapt and overcome; I had been adamant that there would be no improvising or adapting, but that was exactly what I needed to do. To successfully go back to being the person I used to be, I would *have* to improvise and adapt – be less rigid in my thinking.

When I look back through some social media posts I shared at that time, I wonder what on earth was going through my mind. I think I was just desperately trying to prove to myself that I was the same adventurous person I had always been, if not more so; that surgery hadn't taken any part of me away. I certainly enjoyed people's shock and amazement at my latest daring escapade, and that encouraged me to raise the stakes even further. The reality was that it was only ever going to be self-destructive, in one way or another. I had to learn to be like bamboo – patient, strong and flexible. At the moment I was a stick – rigid, dry and liable to snap. I needed to invest in my resilience and not be so terrified of bending every once in a while, as and when required. I needed to adjust my perception of failure, to understand that one rough battle did not mean I'd lost the war. I needed to channel those feelings of anger and frustration into a more productive purpose. I began to find out the hard way that only by doing this would I have any chance of coming back stronger than ever.

CHAPTER 7

It was early September 2019 when we returned to Chamonix. There were mixed emotions, as the previous year I had flown home from Geneva airport feeling upset, disappointed, annoyed and frustrated with myself, for so many reasons. I was still angry that a stupid lump in my head had messed up my life so much. I wondered if I would ever be able to look at the mountains in the same way again. Completing the Yorkshire Three Peaks Challenge had given me a much-needed confidence boost, though, and I began to realise that I was physically able to push myself further than I had previously been able to, which meant I was making progress. OK, it may not have been as swift as I wanted, but progress is progress. Also, I had less reason to fear the potential post-surgery complications, as the risk of those decreased over time. On top of this, Doubt wasn't as much of a familiar face as he had been; he was still around, but not as often.

Unfortunately, on this trip we weren't blessed with the usual sunshine. By the time we arrived, temperatures had dropped about 15 degrees from what they had been the previous week, and the clear skies were now replaced with heavy, leaden clouds. Indeed, the forecast for the duration of our stay was pretty grim.

Chamonix is an outdoor-lovers' paradise. We left our belongings at the hotel and headed off to check out the local shops, as we needed to buy new karabiners, ropes, etc., and I wanted to see if I could remember the French vocab for the things we needed too. It could have been quite disastrous! We ducked in and out of shops trying to avoid the rain, but it was hopeless, and a few hours later we admitted defeat and returned to our room. We were drenched, but at least we had new gear.

As in previous years, we had pre-planned several routes we wanted to cover during our time away. I had also discovered some via ferrata routes in the valley. These are protected climbing routes that employ steel cables, ladders or rungs fixed to the rock. To climb these routes, you wear a harness and two leashes (lanyard) with a braking mechanism that you clip on to the metal fixtures, to limit the drop distance of any falls. Hopefully this wouldn't need to be tested!

I was eager to get out exploring new places and experiences, and with a renewed enthusiasm, all thoughts of possible physical limitations were pushed to the back of my mind. The previous week, I had managed to find online a local mountain guide, Jean, who agreed to lead us on a via ferrata route just outside Chamonix. So, with one eye fixed firmly on the forecast, we arranged for him to collect us early on Saturday morning and drive us to La Curalla at Passy.

Friday was wet and miserable. Mist hung low in the valley, and visibility was poor, as were the conditions on the summits. We decided on a low-level route that day, taking in the cool autumn air, the evergreens of the lower mountain slopes and the distinctive red caps of the fly agaric mushrooms against the moist, fertile, brown earth. Where our route was exposed, through the trees we could just make out the snow-capped mountains of the Mont Blanc Massif, through breaks in the cloud. True to form, I found the steeper sections of our route challenging, but I paced myself, letting Neil go on ahead, comforting myself with the thought that I'd be tired out and I would sleep well that night.

That evening, we laid our gear out and checked it all over, before heading to bed. I lay there, thinking about the challenge we had planned for the following day. My mind was in utter turmoil. I've had some pretty brilliant ideas in the past, but this... well this certainly was beginning to feel as though it wasn't one of them. True to form, just when I needed a good night's sleep, it didn't happen. I clock-watched throughout the night, as each hour passed by. I was tired from our walk anyway and now exhausted with overthinking a particular section of the via ferrata route that would involve crossing a steel cable bridge. I felt sick as I catastrophised in my mind, visualising each precarious step across it and what could go wrong. I really am my own worst enemy at times. None of my coping mechanisms worked that night.

The alarm went off early the following morning, although I was still awake at that time. We got up, showered, and ate the croissants and yogurt we had bought for breakfast. I then spent an hour heading back and forth to the bathroom, as despite my best efforts, Doubt and his friend Nerves had turned up for the event. Marvellous! I was furious and disappointed with myself because I'd worked myself up into such a state the night before, I'd ruined the sleep I so badly needed, and consequently put myself at a greater disadvantage. I was also annoyed that I'd not come up with the idea of doing this before I got ill. Regret can be a consuming and dangerous thing; I think this is one of the things that has led to my new attitude and drive, that feeling of never knowing what lies ahead and how it will affect your plans. That reminder of your own mortality and that we don't always have time ahead of us. Now, more than ever, I wanted to live life to the fullest, but I felt that my efforts to do this were constantly hampered by the effects of my now evicted tumour.

We waited outside for Jean to arrive, but not before I made one last dash back to the bathroom. A white minibus pulled up, and the driver beckoned us over. We jumped in, stowing our rucksacks in the footwell. Jean came across as a quiet but friendly character, his face weathered from the time spent outdoors, and you could tell that he'd had lots of experience of life. He spoke little English, and Neil's French was limited to ordering coffee and pain au chocolat, and so conversation and translation were left to me – with my one good ear!

It was impossible not to notice that he was missing all his fingers from the first joint on each hand, and yet he could still drive. At this point, I'm ashamed to say that I had all sorts of thoughts racing through my mind. This would be my first post-op climb, in an area I wasn't familiar with, and the person I'd enlisted to guide us, who I was trusting with my life, had no fingers. How on earth do you work with ropes and karabiners when you have no fingers or thumbs? Whilst I was reluctant to be intrusive, Neil made it clear that he wanted to know what had happened. It transpires that Jean had a survival story all of his own. If I remember rightly, many years earlier, Jean had been climbing on Mont Blanc. The weather had turned and in a freak accident, he caught his foot in his rope, fell off the rock face, and was left dangling upside down. The plunging temperatures took their toll on his suspended body, and frostbite soon set in. Jean explained that despite losing his fingers, he was determined to continue climbing, and so he taught himself how to do it. He still climbs with friends but does the via ferrata routes on his own. A kindred spirit.

We took half an hour's drive out of town, up into what felt like the middle of nowhere. Once parked up, we put on our harnesses and helmets before beginning our ascent through the woods towards La Curalla, the rock face we would be climbing. I shoved a prochlorperazine tablet down my throat as we walked, and tried to think only about how great it would feel to have achieved this. I was a nervous wreck, but turning back at that point was not an option for me.

116

As we arrived at the rock face, Jean tied on the rope. Yes, you heard me right. The man with so little in the way of fingers tied us all on to the rope. It was impressive to watch, as his short stumps tied knots and opened and closed karabiners with ease. My admiration for him grew with every second. He patiently explained to me how to clip on and off each section, how to make sure the rope was tensioned correctly, and so on, and I relayed the instructions back to Neil in English. Jean led the way and took the first step, followed by Neil, and I went last…

That first step was nerve-wracking. My heart was pounding so loudly in my chest, I'm surprised no one else could hear it. From that point on, I was so fixated on what I had to do that Nerves didn't get a look in. Each step, each handhold, each clip on and off of the lanyard, and each rope fixing. Time seemed to stand still. This is what being in the zone is all about.

All thoughts of that cable bridge section had slipped my mind until I came around one outcrop to suddenly be faced with it. There was no exit strategy at this point; the only way was across it. As I took my first tentative step onto the steel cable, I looked ahead towards Neil, rather than down, knowing there were hundreds of metres of nothing between me and the cloud that was clinging to the rock like a mystical cloak. Ahead of me, some small alpine plants were growing out of tiny cracks in the rock. Unintentionally holding my breath, I focussed on a small bit of greenery and carefully took my first few steps. I could feel the rope swaying beneath me as I moved. Cautiously, I grasped the cable that ran along my right side at shoulder height, trying to slide my gloved hand along without leaning into it, as I knew that if my balance failed and I was to fall there, I'd be waiting for a rescue team to come and get me. I could never live through the embarrassment of that, the inconvenience to everyone, or the spoiling of Neil's day. Slowly, I inched my way across the steel cable, until I reached Jean and Neil on the other side. I took a deep breath, my heart still pounding away. I'd done it.

Once across, we then climbed up to a narrow ridge. At least, Neil told me there was a ridge there to step on to. From the position I was climbing to it from, I couldn't see what was beneath me. Sure enough, the rock ledge was there, and we stopped briefly and took in what little views we had, as the cloud hung in the valley below us. As we continued our upwards climb, I lost all track of time. Eventually, the rock became interspersed with tree roots and loose soil, and finally grass. We had made it. I pulled myself up the final section and onto the gravelly path. At this point, I was able to take a deep breath and finally revel in my latest achievement.

Taking off our helmets, ropes and harnesses, we began our descent, this time via a steep woodland path. At least, it seemed steep to me; Jean was nimble on his feet, almost running downhill, whilst for me each step on the stony ground was precarious. Every move was thought out, ensuring that there was a tree or rock I could aim for, to stop myself if gravity got the better of me. By comparison, the climb up that I had been so nervous about now seemed to be easy. Neil and Jean had reached the minibus long before I had made it down. There was a small wooden hut nearby that hired out equipment, as well as selling snacks and drinks. Jean knew the people who owned the place, and they treated us all to well-deserved ice cream and drinks! They were wonderful. We chatted about where we were from and had the chance of a quick cuddle with their lovely, elderly dog before Jean drove us back to Chamonix.

It had been such an amazing experience, and one that could easily have not happened if I'd have let my fears stop me. I have on many occasions concluded that stepping out of our comfort zones is the best way of building resilience. With each challenge, I was not only becoming physically stronger, but mentally tougher too. I was beginning to understand that many battles are won in the mind. They are won by those who admit their areas of weakness to themselves, and work to understand them; why they happen, how they happen, and what the impact is; those who sit and think about them, working out strategies to improve. They are won by those who attend to the detail, chipping away, building their confidence, and overcoming every obstacle, because they know they can, and will not entertain failure.

Leaving Chamonix this time around was a different experience. The fears, disappointments and doubts about the previous trip had been banished and I now felt triumphant. The only thing that had scuppered some of our plans this year was the weather, not me and my potential inadequacies. Now, as we headed home, my head was full of plans for the future. I'm not sure how Doubt and Nerves made it back, but they weren't with me.

CHAPTER 8

It was about a week after our return to the UK when I received a text message from my friend Cerries, who was off to climb Toubkal, a mountain peak in southwestern Morocco, at the end of the month. A few months earlier, whilst we were out hiking, I had jokingly said to her that if she were to change her mind, or wanted to smuggle me in a holdall, I would happily go along! You know that expression 'be careful what you wish for…'; her message read something along the lines of, "You jokingly said about coming to Toubkal. One of the girls broke her hand yesterday when we were training on the Watkin path in Snowdonia. Would you be interested in joining the trip?"

Initially, I hesitated. There were all manner of things to consider. I had commitments in the studio, tuition work booked in, and more worryingly, nothing in the way of savings to finance the trip. But with a few more messages received from Cerries saying, "Tempting isn't it?" and "Come on, the highest mountain in North Africa awaits you…", I really wanted to go and knew that I would regret it forever if I didn't; I asked the question "How much?" It was more reasonable than I expected and, more importantly, it was within reach. It didn't take much for me to make my decision. There were, of course, a few logistics to sort out; ticket names needed to be changed, insurance for high altitude to be organised and a few extra bits of gear to buy, but with just two weeks' notice, I managed to get together everything I needed and I was ready to head off to Morocco.

A week before our departure, we met up with Gwyn, himself an accomplished mountaineer, medic and former mountain rescue team member, who would be travelling with us. I also met Jay, who was the reason the trip was taking place, as he missed out on the climb the previous year, having been taken ill upon arrival at Marrakech. Cerries had asked me to bring a list of any medical conditions and medications with me. As I presented Gwyn with an A4 sheet detailing my medical history and medication list, I felt physically sick, half expecting him not to allow me on the trip. Why would anyone want a liability like me tagging along? How wrong I was. He seemed completely undaunted, and I did wonder if this was a good or bad thing; I didn't want to consider what he might be thinking and had decided not to say. Over dinner that evening, we discussed the itinerary for the trip, flight details, transfer from the airport, and the support crew we would have with us, as well as some local customs and behaviours for us to observe whilst in Morocco.

So, on Saturday 28th September we would fly out from Manchester to Marrakech. From there we would be transported to Matat village at 1,850 m, where we would spend our first night. The following day, we would hike up to 3,000 m before dropping back down to Refuge de la Tazarhart at 2,970 m, where we would spend the night before continuing the following morning to base camp – Toubkal refuge at 3,200 m. On Tuesday 1st October, we would have a very early wake-up call and head for the summit at 4,167 m, before heading back to base camp. The following day, after summiting, we would descend through the valley to the village of Sidi Chamharouch at 2,310 m, where we would rest for a few hours before continuing to Aroumd village, where we would stay overnight. There we would say goodbye to our support team before finally heading back to Marrakech for a few days of rest and relaxation before flying home the following Saturday.

One of our biggest problems was going to be the possibility of AMS (acute mountain sickness, often referred to as altitude sickness), which usually occurs from around 2,400 m; Toubkal is 4,167 m. At that altitude, both oxygen levels and air pressure are noticeably lower than at sea level; the oxygen level is around 60% of what it is at sea level, and although the human body can adapt, sometimes, especially if your body is under the sort of exertion that is required for mountain climbing, it can't adapt quickly enough. AMS can just hit you, with no warning. The symptoms are both many and varied; in mild cases it can be dizziness, headache, muscle aches, insomnia, nausea and vomiting, nose bleeds, irritability, loss of appetite, swelling of the hands, feet and face, rapid heartbeat and shortness of breath. However, in more severe cases, it can be coughing, chest congestion, discolouration or paleness of skin, inability to walk, lack of balance and social withdrawal. There are some factors that increase your chances of getting it: living at sea level, quick movement from low to high altitudes, the physical exertion involved, extreme heights, a low red blood cell count due to anaemia, heart or lung disease, medications such as sleeping pills, painkillers or tranquillisers or past bouts of severe AMS. Generally, for most people, it's quite mild and will clear up, but it can cause brain and/or lung issues for some. Now, I already ticked a number of boxes on that list, and I didn't know if it would increase the severity of my symptoms, or just allow everyone else to feel the same as I do every day – it was an unknown quantity.

In preparation for the possibility of AMS, it had been planned for us to adopt a strategy of 'climb high and sleep low', giving our bodies the best opportunity to adapt to the lower oxygen levels and air pressure during two separate 24 hour periods. We would be climbing over 1,000 m each day, so that sounded like a very good plan indeed.

The reality of it all was beginning to dawn on me; this was huge. A seriously huge mountain. In the middle of nowhere. As far as post-op achievements go, this would be monumental. I was so very excited, yet nervous as hell too.

The night before I was due to fly, I barely slept a wink. I woke up feeling exhausted, my tinnitus louder than it had ever been, and pulsating so loudly down my ear that at times it actually became painful. A great start – not. I double checked I had everything and weighed my holdall once again. It was over the limit. I cried and unpacked, throwing everything onto my bed, unable to logically think about what to leave behind. I might need all of it. Wondering what the commotion was, Neil came upstairs to find me having a meltdown, so he calmly told me to relax, took hold of the kit list, and together we went through every single item: first-aid kit, that was in; camera equipment, that made the cut; one pair of trousers, taken out; a t-shirt out; buff out; hat replaced with lighter cap; and so on… Finally, now within the weight limit, we locked the bag up.

Neil drove me to meet up with Cerries and Gwyn, before Jay drove us all to the airport. I had cried all morning; I felt so emotionally torn between wanting to go and staying home, where I was safe. I gave myself every possible reason not to go; since my surgery, I struggled with airports, because of the noise and the sheer volume of people. I was so worried about not travelling with Neil, as he knew me well and recognised when I was finding things tough. I felt incredibly underprepared because of the short notice. Doubt reappeared and asked a few questions… What if I couldn't keep up because of my fatigue? What if I slipped and injured myself? What would medical facilities be like there? What if I struggled with the altitude? What if… What if… What if? Running through all of this though, was another question – What if I could actually do this?

As we began our final approach to Marrakech airport, we could clearly see the city, lit up by beautiful, colourful lights.

Cerries and I smiled to ourselves, as a young woman sat directly behind us, commented about how surprised she was that the Christmas lights (Morocco is a Muslim country) were up already… The weather forecast for our trip looked perfect but incredibly hot. On the day of our arrival, temperatures had reached the mid-40s and as we disembarked from our aircraft, we were instantly hit by an incredible wall of dry heat. We made our way through passport control, immigration checks, and finally collected our luggage. Thankfully, it had all arrived, although I'd packed some essentials in my rucksack just in case anything had gone amiss, so that we could at least start our trek as planned.

Our local organiser, Ibrahim, and his friend were waiting to greet us outside the airport building; in fact, he should have been our guide for the trip but had injured his ankle a few days earlier whilst running down Toubkal's scree slopes, with a team of Australians. They were both so friendly and welcoming. Our bags were loaded onto the roof of the Land Cruiser, lashed securely on with rope, and we were handed some very welcome bottles of chilled water. We began our journey, away from the bright lights of the city and out into the middle of nowhere. Leaving the main road, we eventually headed upwards on rocky tracks. We seemed perilously close to the edge of the mountainside; the sharp hairpin bends began to get tighter and tighter until the driver had to stop, back up, and take the bend in two or more attempts. I was glad not to have a window seat! In the dark, we could barely see our surroundings but I imagined the hillsides to be red and sandy. We could make out odd piles of pallet boxes ready for harvesting apples.

As our vehicle headed deeper into the mountains, we reached the point where we ran out of road and had to make the rest of the journey on foot. We were guided by two men, who had been waiting for us, flashing torches in the distance. When we reached them, they unloaded our large holdalls and in no time disappeared, carrying them up ahead. I fumbled through my rucksack in the dark, looking for a torch, which to my horror I soon realised was in my holdall. I was struggling with staying upright in the total darkness we now found ourselves in, and so I had to make do with the light from my phone. I was tired from sitting so long, and now I was expecting my remaining vestibular system to suddenly wake up and walk on rough ground, in the dark. I could easily have scuppered my chances of summiting there and then! As I took a deep breath, I looked up to be greeted by a sky full of stars, too many to count, and a picture book view of the milky way high above us. It was utterly breathtaking, just knowing that each of those stars was as big, or even bigger than our star, the sun. At that moment, staring up at the illuminated sky, I knew that I was ready to do this.

Following Ibrahim, who despite hobbling along wearing flip-flops over his poorly bandaged foot, was still able to move quicker than me in the dark, the four of us made our way along narrow, rocky paths cut into the hillside until we reached a deserted-looking building. It seemed to be a big house, but it was in total darkness. The first door we went to was locked, so following behind Ibrahim, like a clutch of chicks behind their mother, we made our way back around to the other side of the building, where the door was open. We were led by our hosts along a narrow, tiled hallway into another room with two long sofas either side and a low table down the centre, laid out ready for us to eat. We were presented with huge tagines full of stew, cous-cous, and the most vibrantly coloured salad, as well as refreshing, sugar-loaded mint tea. It was delicious.

I was tired and struggling to keep my stinging eyes open. It was around 1:00 a.m. by the time we got to bed. Our rooms were clean but very basic. We had a narrow bed each; Cerries' was up against the wall opposite the door and mine was adjacent to the window. The window itself had no panes of glass, just shutters between us and the outside world. The toilet (some walk away) was a malodorous long drop, with no lock on the door and a bucket of water with which to flush. We freshened up in a wash-basin outside our room, each of us taking turns to keep lookout for the other. It was certainly basic, but I was more than ready to embrace this simplistic, no-frills way of life for the next week. It was part of the deal.

That first night was stifling, and with the wooden shutters closed, there was no breeze at all, so I just lay on top of my opened sleeping bag. I was so tired, I soon drifted off. Surprisingly, I slept well that night, waking early the following morning for breakfast. We ate in the same room as the previous night; this time we were warmly welcomed with an enormous pot of porridge, teas, coffee, freshly baked bread, honey, cheeses and meats. We all tucked in, knowing we would be needing every drop of energy for the long day that lay ahead of us. I took my 'dizzy pills' and sorted out my camera equipment, before packing away the rest of my gear and carrying my holdall up the stone staircase to where our support team were ready and waiting, to load up the mules. We would just be wearing a day sack, carrying our own essentials from water and snacks to hats, sun cream and first-aid kit.

Outside on the terrace, I was now able to see for the first time the mysterious village we had arrived in the night before. The building in which we had spent the night, along with the others in the village, was built from brick that looked as though it had been crudely cut from rock. Cream paint framed each window aperture, the openings filled with an ornate powder-blue grill. The roof, along with those of all the other buildings that I could see, appeared to be a basic but functional concrete slab. Nothing more than shutters would keep out the elements of this harsh mountain environment. This seemed to be the most complete and decorated house in the area. Others looked like they were still in the process of being built; there were no shutters, and some appeared to have no roofs. Laundry, hung out to dry between houses, fluttered in the warm breeze, and small children could be heard laughing somewhere nearby.

The views from our terrace were spectacular. There were resplendent mountains as far as I could see, just waiting to be explored. The merciless sun, which hadn't yet reached its apex, cast shadows down the mountain slopes, the darkness hanging in ravines and gullies, resembling swathes of inky-dark velvet. The lower slopes were dotted with shrubs and olive trees, like flecks of ink on a blank manuscript. In the distance, fertile green terraces used for farming were cut deep into the land, contrasting brightly with the brown dusty-looking earth; above, jagged peaks were silhouetted against the azure blue sky, whilst down below, chickens roamed freely on the rocky paths, with the sound of a cockerel and some mules carried towards us on the gentle breeze. Excitement coursed through my veins; it was so very good to be alive.

After a final check of our gear, we were ready to go. Led by our guide, Lahcen, who the previous night had run (yes, run) from the next village to meet us, we set off, followed a short time later by our mules, who were carrying our holdalls and supplies. It was hot, around 40 degrees, but it was a bearable dry heat, which does make a difference. Gwyn was soon on our case reminding us to keep sipping water, as that would help with fatigue and any effects of altitude, as well as the obvious dehydration. The scenery was stunning, and the rocky paths were quiet. When we stood still, there was nothing but blissful silence. How I loved the solitude of these mountains.

Once we left the protective shelter that the village afforded us, we were exposed. There was no shade as the blazing sun beat down on us. We took a short break in the shade of a couple of olive trees, as my hearing aid battery had decided that was the perfect moment to go flat. It was so wonderfully peaceful. In the distance, an elderly man, stooped with age, was heading towards us, his mule carrying his belongings. He gave us a toothless smile and waved as he passed by, and soon after, we too continued on our way.

Whilst only in his early twenties, our local guide Lahcen confidently told us that he had summited Toubkal many times, the first time being with his father when he was just 12 years old. He was an affable character, always smiling, laughing, and singing western songs whilst adding his own Berber influence and sway, as we made our way higher into the mountains. His equipment was basic and well worn, and he would refill his empty coke bottle with the chilled, crystal clear water that flowed down from the mountains. "Okie dokie!" he would say, as we moved on. The rest of us would echo him. Gwyn was soon known affectionately as 'Ali Baba', and as Lahcen called out "You OK Ali Baba?" to Gwyn, who had taken up the position of last man, Gwyn would reply, "Yes, Super Berberman!"

Along our route, we came upon a small stall that had been set up on the side of the hill. An elderly gentleman offered us freshly pressed orange juice and mint tea. He had connected up his own chilled water supply straight from the mountain stream, and this was used not only for making the tea but also to keep cool the oranges and other drinks he was selling. It was such a simplistic setup, yet pure genius. We sat down under the crudely made shade, whilst he placed a tray of mint tea on a low table, made from what looked like a plastic milk crate with an old fridge door balanced precariously on top of it. It did the job.

What really struck me was how happy Lahcen, and the other people we met along our way, were. They had none of the luxuries we often crave and are accustomed to, their lives were comparably simplistic, and yet everyone whose path we crossed was smiling, happy and content. They all helped each other, too. This will stay with me for a long time, and I'm certain that there is a lesson to be learned there.

We stopped for a while to watch the misadventure of some goats play out before our eyes. Lahcen had heard rocks falling, and it transpired that some mountain goats were kicking them down at us, seeing us as a threat. Nearby, another small group of goats had ventured down the steep, perilous mountainside onto some rocky outcrops, where grass was growing. It looked as though one of them, who had clearly gorged himself on the vegetation growing on the small outcrop he'd claimed, had over-indulged to the extent he was now struggling to get back up. We stayed awhile, waiting to see the fate of this poor goat that had become stuck, but eventually we had to move on as we were losing time. Thinking back to the many National Geographic documentaries I have watched of goats and other mountainous animals scrambling up and down seemingly impossible terrain, I hoped this particular little goat's story would have a similar happy ending.

Halfway through our day's journey, we stopped beside a waterfall. From seemingly nowhere, Lahcen produced fresh bread rolls, sardines, oranges and nuts for us all. It was not the kind of packed lunch I would normally have brought out for a day's hiking, but it certainly did the job. Having rested, rehydrated and refuelled, we were ready to continue climbing uphill to our next stop.

After a few hours more walking, Refuge de la Tazarhart appeared in the distance, at first as a small, easy-to-miss blot on the barren, rocky landscape. We climbed a little higher towards the ridge, before then dropping down to the basic building at 2,970 m altitude. We arrived ahead of the mules, so once we had descended the scree path down to the perfectly camouflaged small stone building, we put down our day sacks and poles, and after a few minutes of stretching out our aching limbs, we headed inside to explore.

The refuge was a deceptive building, small on the outside, large on the inside – almost Tardis-like. We entered through a narrow hallway used for equipment storage into a fairly decent-sized dining area. Cooking equipment was basic, with meals being prepared on hobs fitted to gas bottles along the left-hand wall, which faced out towards the valley we had just walked along. There was a mezzanine sleeping area at the far end of the room, where around six guides could sleep, whilst we were told we would sleep on the next level, in the roof space. We climbed up the ladder, past the mezzanine floor, and into the roof, dragging our holdalls and day sacks with us. Up there, there were around 20 mattresses lined up on either side, in the eaves. That day there would just be the four of us, our team and a Spanish couple with their guide, who arrived later.

Down below, our team worked hard to prepare meals and supplies for us. Once we had set up our sleeping space, we came back down to snack on freshly made popcorn and mint tea. The refuge was about as basic as you could get. Wash facilities were at the kitchen sink, and so personal hygiene, washing in front of the Berber guides, wouldn't really have been appropriate; wet wipes, hand sanitiser and dry wash became our friends, and valuable commodities. We nicknamed the toilet, 'the loo with a view'. A rather precarious rocky path led down to the toilet; it was quite literally cut into rock below the building, a wooden door bolted to the entrance. Should you have unfortunately made a wrong turn, there was quite a considerable drop. This was another fragrant long drop, complete with a water tap (piped in from the mountain stream) and bucket to flush with. There was a small diamond-shaped hole in the top of the door to let in light and air. However, it also meant you would be on full view to anyone who happened to be waiting outside, so my versatile shemagh (a traditional Arabian scarf) soon became my privacy screen, as I crudely hung it from a nail above the door. There was no lighting, so at that point, despite protests from Gwyn, we collectively made the conscious decision to reduce our fluid intake, so we wouldn't need to make a precarious visit during the night!

We invited our guide and muleteers to eat the main evening meal with us, but they politely declined. Once we had finished eating, our crew ate their meals made up from what we had left,

131

which seemed to be so unfair, as they were working far harder than we were: looking after the mules, carrying our gear around, and cooking with the most basic of equipment – we tried our hardest, but we couldn't sway them. After another mouth-watering meal, followed by 'sleepy tea', we sat down to discuss our plan for the following day, going over each detail of the route and the equipment we would need to be carrying on us.

Whilst the team below were laying out their prayer mats, we made our last evening trip to the loo with a view. Outside, the sun was setting behind the jagged peaks, either side of the valley, and I watched on as the orange hues became darkness, the temperature noticeably dropped and a cool breeze picked up in the valley. The flickering stars once again began to reveal themselves. My balance being what it is in the dark, I headed inside to bed as soon as night fell.

It was a disturbed sleep that night; it felt as though Doubt had made the journey up the valley on the mules and caught up with me. My anxiety levels hadn't been helped by the fact I was unable to speak to Neil that day, as we were well away from any network coverage; I hadn't realised how much I needed the comfort of hearing his voice. That evening, the guides staying with us in the refuge had all placed their phones up against the glass of the window, celebrating each time they managed to make some sort of connection. It was fun to watch, but at that moment I would have given anything to call home.

I woke the next morning, feeling as tired as I had when I went to bed, with a cacophony of sound pulsating somewhere deep in the left side of my head. How I wished I could just switch it off, and get some respite from the drone. After a wonderful carb- and protein-loaded breakfast, we headed outside to clean our teeth in some purified water that Gwyn had set aside for us. Our journey to Toubkal base camp began early. The air was cool, as the sun's powerful rays hadn't yet made their way into the depths of the valley.

What had been a fairly easy descent down from the ridge to the refuge the previous day now became a more precarious, slippery, exposed climb out of the valley on loose gravel and scree. My poles were a godsend, and as time went on, I found myself using them not just to dig in and pull myself along, but also as a means of creating more spatial awareness, allowing me to move a little faster than I would have done otherwise. Lahcen appeared to be able to pick a pace that suited us all, and as planned we began our trek up towards the top of the valley. It wasn't long before we reached the infamous zigzags that Cerries had previously told me about. It was one of the main routes into the next valley, and apparently there were a hundred of them. After the distraction of having to move out of the way for a couple of oncoming mules to pass, and Lahcen singing a Berber version of *Africa* by Shakira, keeping count of the hairpin bends became an impossible task. By the time we reached the top of the valley, it certainly felt like there could've been a hundred twists and turns, if not more.

It was going to be a long day. The emotion of the days leading to our departure, the sensory overload at the airport, and not sleeping in my own bed, not to mention the apprehension about our summit day, were all beginning to take their toll. Doubt floated alongside me, pulling faces, taunting me. Having completed the zigzags, we took a break. By this point, I was really starting to feel fatigued, but I carried on. At around 3,600 m, and just before we began our descent once more towards base camp, we had another rest stop, which had come not a moment too soon; I had pushed on, not wanting anyone to notice that I was struggling. If I'd been alone, I think I might have found myself a sheltered spot and slept for an hour to recuperate. Again, Lahcen rustled up a small meal for us: bread, sardines, boiled eggs and nuts followed by slices of orange. We perched ourselves down on the rocks and refuelled. It was from this rest stop that we caught our first sight of Toubkal. It seemed so distant and out of reach, yet this time tomorrow we'd be on the summit.

About an hour before we reached base camp, we dropped down into the next valley to be greeted by our muleteer and cook, who had created the most amazing tagine meal you could ever imagine. How they managed to prepare this amazing feast with nothing more than a gas bottle and just a few utensils, is beyond me. A long mat and cushioned seating had been laid out for us on the mountainside, and we sat down, as Lahcen poured the tea into small glasses. Our meal, some sort of chickpea stew served up with brightly coloured fresh salad and couscous, was delicious, and very much needed by this point. We sat eating and drinking freshly brewed mint tea, overlooking the valley with base camp just visible as a dot in the distance. Whilst we rested, cloud rolled through the valley below. As the dark, ominous veil passed through, we watched on as rain fell, continuing out of sight towards Imlil village with thankfully just a few drops of rain reaching us on the gentle, warm breeze.

By this point, I was beginning to tire and was suffering from nosebleeds, apparently not unusual at altitude, although they could also have been caused by the amount of dust in the air. I had developed a slight headache that felt slightly different from the usual ones, like a pressure band across my forehead, but it was tolerable; taking a couple of paracetamol and increasing the amount of water I was drinking seemed to help, as it soon eased off. I was worried that if I mentioned this to Gwyn he'd tell me I couldn't summit, but once I did open up and confess, he was great and nothing but supportive.

We continued down into the valley, along narrow and exposed paths. I was glad to reach base camp, as it had been an arduous day. Totally remote, in this barren landscape, Les Mouflons Refuge, another stone building, blended in perfectly with its surroundings. It was a micro village, or compound, deep in the middle of nowhere with its own unique atmosphere and sense of camaraderie, particularly amongst the guides, who all seemed to know each other and were pleased to meet up, with handshaking, back slapping and sharing jovial jokes. We were shown to our dormitory, a long dark room with a small window at the far end. Along each side were bunks, with mattresses lined up side by side on two levels. Cerries and I bagged our spot and put our sleeping bags out to claim our territory. There was shelving at our end near the door, so the bags, boots and poles were stored there, and next door was a proper toilet, showers and washbasin with a cold tap – bliss!

Lahcen called us over for the tea and biscuits that had been prepared for us. Then, fortunately having managed to find enough 3G coverage to finally make a call to Neil, I stood on the terrace in the late afternoon sun, overlooking the campsite, where mules roamed freely. I shared the events of the day, how spectacular the scenery was, and just how wonderful our team were. Speaking to him provided a confidence boost, and once we ended our call I headed off to bed for a much-needed nap. It wasn't much longer until Cerries turned in too. I lay there listening to music as people of all nationalities came and went, but I was unable to block out the roaring tinnitus in my head. We ate well that night at the refuge and prepared our gear ready for the next morning, as we planned to leave early. The Camelbak water reservoir was filled, first-aid kit and tablets put in, coat, extra layers, gloves, hat, sunglasses… in it all went. The day sack was heavier than it had been in previous days, as we had to be prepared for both heat and cold.

I went to bed that night, feeling a mixture of apprehension and excitement for our summit day. It was well after midnight before I finally drifted off into a fitful sleep, dreaming about the goal I had wanted to fulfil for so long. Unfortunately, we were woken at 3:00 a.m., when the French contingent who were sharing the room decided to get up and get their gear ready in the dorm, with little consideration for everyone else. Trying to think of suitable expletives in a foreign language on three hours' sleep, even though I knew a few, wasn't easy; I think I managed it, though. I lay there with my eyes tightly shut, behind my eye mask until 5:00 a.m., hoping that rest would be just as good as sleep, then got up and slipped into my gear that I'd left prepared at the end of my mattress. I had taken one of Neil's tops, and had decided to wear that as I was really missing him, and wanted to feel like he was in some way with me for this incredible day. I headed down for another hearty breakfast of porridge, 'Berber pancakes' and several cups of coffee.

The first section of our ascent out of base camp was a little bit of a scramble, with just the light of our head torches showing us the way. Again, this was difficult for me, but I'd done it before and this wasn't going to stop me. With Lahcen leading the way, we hit the scree slopes just as the sun began to rise, silhouetting the high mountains around us. It was a beautiful sight, and we paused to take it in. As we stood there looking across the valley, the mountains turned a beautiful orange and the sky a vivid blue. The silence was broken only by the distant rumble of falling rocks.

The scree slopes were, as expected, tough for me. At times, it felt like I was trying to stay upright whilst walking on ball bearings. Gwyn likened it to marbles on lino! My poles were great for digging in and giving me that extra bit of contact with the ground. We passed a number of other teams who had made an early start and were now coming down from the summit, as we clawed our way upwards on the scree. Many of them had ascended for sunrise on the summit, but there were so many of them, it must have been like a superhighway up there. Taking frequent breaks for water, and to take a look around at just how far we had come, we made steady progress. The scree path became rockier and steeper as we made our way up the final ascent, before levelling off. We had made good time that morning, reaching the summit by 10:30 a.m. Gwyn had explained the route to me, describing how the path seemed to take a final turn back on itself, before you see the steel pyramid structure at the top. I was up in front with Lahcen, who seemed to understand just how much this meant to me. Once we made that final hairpin turn, he stepped aside to let me see the summit first, on my own. I will always be so grateful for that.

I don't think I will ever be able to explain the emotion of that moment, how seeing the summit pyramid against the deep blue sky made me feel. Up ahead of me, it was so near and yet appeared so far. What had once seemed unreachable was now there, almost within touching distance. My mind flashed back to the images I had looked at on the internet and in magazines; they just didn't do it justice. I thought of how for so long I had wanted to come here and how it had seemed to be an impossible dream. Now here I was, and there was the summit, almost within my grasp. My breathing quickened uncontrollably as the emotion began to set in, and behind my sunglasses, I fought back tears from the one eye that can still cry. I felt so emotional. I was so ecstatic to be here, but there was a tinge of sadness, as the one person I wanted more than anything to share this experience with was thousands of miles away.

I had an uncontrollable urge to reach the summit, and from nowhere found the energy to pick up my pace. The others were a couple of minutes behind, but when they reached the top we hugged, we cried and we took in the most incredible views over the Sahara and the vast Atlas mountain range. At that moment, we were the highest human beings in North Africa. As far as the eye could see, there was ridge after ridge of mountains, resembling crests of waves in a sea of rock; the peaks glinting in the sunlight, the troughs casting mysterious shadows. Looking out towards the horizon, our view of this Martian-like landscape became obscured by a thin veil of mist. There are no words to describe what it means to achieve a goal that so many times I thought would be impossible. I spent a few minutes unable to speak, just wanting to savour every single moment of my time on the summit, not wanting to leave this experience, this feeling of accomplishment, behind.

I busied myself taking photos, wanting to capture every single moment to look back on in years to come, whilst Lahcen prepared our food. Again, out of his bag, he produced boiled eggs, sardines, bread rolls, oranges and nuts. It had been a long morning and we would be needing this for the tricky, arduous hike back down. It was superb. For me, this had been so much more than an adventure. It had been a dream come true. A dream I had once thought might never be, and one that might never have been had I listened to Doubt. I had come to realise just how much I was still capable of achieving despite the many obstacles I still face. I think I had left Doubt a little way behind, still scrambling on the scree, never to make the summit.

Gwyn told me the following day that he understood just what I had been through, as he had lost his mother – his best friend, a nurse – to a brain tumour. Hearing this identified a new emotion that I had been feeling but didn't understand: survivor guilt. How could life be so cruel to take someone who not only was so obviously loved, but a nurse, who did so much for others, and yet spare me? Once more, I felt guilty that I had survived what others hadn't, and not only survived but achieved incredible things; in just 506 days, I had gone from lying in a hospital, unable to walk, to scaling this summit.

Toubkal had been on my to-do list for such a long time. As it was the first, but hopefully not the last, 'big' climb since surgery, this will always be a special mountain to me and I am so grateful to everyone who made it possible. I love mountains; they are the ultimate metaphor for life. You can't always see the top, but you have to stay committed and keep on pushing, whilst remembering to enjoy the journey along the way. Mountains have an atmosphere like nothing else. I love the peace and solitude that I find in these remote places. I love the silence – since losing my hearing, they are a safe haven where I don't have to worry about noise, and I love the challenges they present.

I feel lucky to still be here; I *am* lucky to still be here, and have made a promise to myself to make every day count for something. I still look for and find those silver linings. Whilst my diagnosis was devastating and life changing, and I wish it had never happened, I feel blessed that it has changed my perspective on life in so many ways; only by going through an experience like that can you ever truly understand, but I hope that I have shown you a little of it.

As we squared away our gear, put our rucksacks back on, and began our treacherous descent down the scree slopes, I had just one thought… What next?

AFTERWORD

It's 8:00 a.m., Saturday 25th July, 2020. A warm, cloudy, humid morning with a forecast of mixed sunshine and showers, and the threat of thunderstorms. I'm feeling happy. I'm feeling confident. I'm about to start running the entire length of the Sandstone Trail, 55 kilometres in length with 1,268 m of ascent; an undulating path following sandstone ridges, made up of 225-million-year old Triassic sandstone. It runs from the ancient market town of Frodsham in Cheshire, to rural Whitchurch in North Shropshire. I've decided to run from south to north, as I will finish closer to home. I cannot wait to begin.

Toubkal. There have been a few bumps in the road since then: some I've handled well and some not so well. 2020 brought a new set of challenges and unprecedented uncertainty for all of us. I returned from Morocco feeling on top of the world (after almost standing on it), but it wasn't long before the empty, bereft post-challenge feeling returned and I was left wondering what I could do next. Sadly, I lost two good friends to cancer, which had a far greater impact than I expected, and actually dabbled with my mental health. I was still making good progress in terms of my physical recovery, but the mental aspect? Nah, not so good. I was suffering with feelings of tremendous guilt, which I didn't understand, as I had so much to be grateful for. My fatigue increased, and Anger and Frustration joined in the party. Apparently, this is absolutely normal, but no one tells you that and you don't expect the wheels to fall off at that stage. Doubt once again became my companion, happily encouraging every negative feeling he could possibly find and revelling in it. My usual coping strategies now began to fail, and I realised that something was seriously wrong.

Calling upon every bit of courage that I had, I contacted Andrea, my specialist nurse. I'm not sure what I expected, whether it be wringing of hands or pulling of hair, but I was surprised by the calm reassurance and understanding, and I realised that she'd seen it all before; she felt that I would benefit from some support from the acquired brain injury team. Doubt told me that I didn't need that sort of help, and I could do this on my own. I ignored him. With their help I have been able to work on fatigue management strategies and restructure my way of thinking. I have talked everything through with my neuropsychologist (impossible at first, floodgates at the end) and made future plans in line with my personal values; although they are very different to my pre-diagnosis plans, they are plans that I'm happy with. The Brain Injury Service has helped me to realise that the way I had been feeling was completely normal. Now, thanks to their input, I feel empowered.

I had so many hopes and dreams for 2020, but the Covid-19 pandemic meant that many of those are now on hold indefinitely, as they are for the majority of us. I needed to find focus. I needed something to give me a new daily purpose and goal.

At the start of the year, I enlisted the help of Jon Fearne, an endurance athlete coach. I hesitantly told him of my plans and received nothing but support and great guidance; he felt that my goals were within reach. I was nervous about working with him; as Doubt pointed out, I'm hardly Paula Radcliffe and I was struggling to complete three 30 minute runs a week, but with Jon's help I soon found myself training five to six days a week, whilst also working on core strength and balance. Quite honestly, I'd never felt better. I cannot emphasize enough just how important it is to surround yourself with people who support you and lift you when you're feeling low.

I continue to advocate for the raising of awareness of brain tumours and hidden disabilities, and take on challenges to fundraise for causes that are close to my heart. I still work in my photography studio, which can be a challenge on the not-so-good days but is still something I very much enjoy. More recently, I have started a slightly different journey, as a grandparent; I'm sure lots of fun and adventures lie ahead with Rico.

So, here I am literally at the start of the latest challenge. My good friend Cerries is planning to meet me at certain points, to spur me on, offer encouragement and route pointers. Neil will join me at roughly the halfway point, just for some moral support. I know it's going to be tough, both mentally and physically, and it will be the furthest I've ever run in my life. I will also be running alone. Just me alone with my thoughts for hours. Is this a good idea? Of course. Will I be capable of it? I think so; no, scratch that. Yes, I am perfectly capable of it.

What would have happened if I'd just accepted the hand that fate had chosen to give to me? If I had accepted the balance issues and lived my life within the anticipated limitations? If I hadn't taken any risks or set goals and worked towards them? Well, I wouldn't be running the Sandstone Trail, that's for sure. Life is all about choices. Whether it's a job you're unhappy in, your health suffering through a poor lifestyle, wanting to increase your fitness, or being in a bad relationship for whatever reason. *You* are the master of your own destiny. *You* can control, direct and influence huge swathes of what happens in your life. *You* can make your life whatever you want it to be. It all begins and ends with *you*.

In addition to my friends and family, I have so many people to thank for helping me to get this far. I have had incredible support from the British Acoustic Neuroma Association (BANA), Brain Tumour Research and Head Injured People (HIP) in Cheshire. If you feel you are struggling (or listening to Doubt), please, please, please ask for help; it's out there, it's brilliant and you won't regret it. The Brain Injury Service has helped me out of my serious rut when I didn't think anything would help, and whilst I've got to be honest and say that Doubt still shows his face from time to time, I don't worry about him now, as I know how to handle him.

I still suffer with the after-effects of my acoustic neuroma, more than I want, less than it could have been. The thing is though, my future is bright. With a few deep breaths and a smile on my face, I start to run...

Printed in Great Britain
by Amazon